Keto Appetizers

Beginner's Guide to Burning Fat, Losing Weight, Lowering Inflammation, and Improving Anxiety & Depression

Sally Alvarez

1

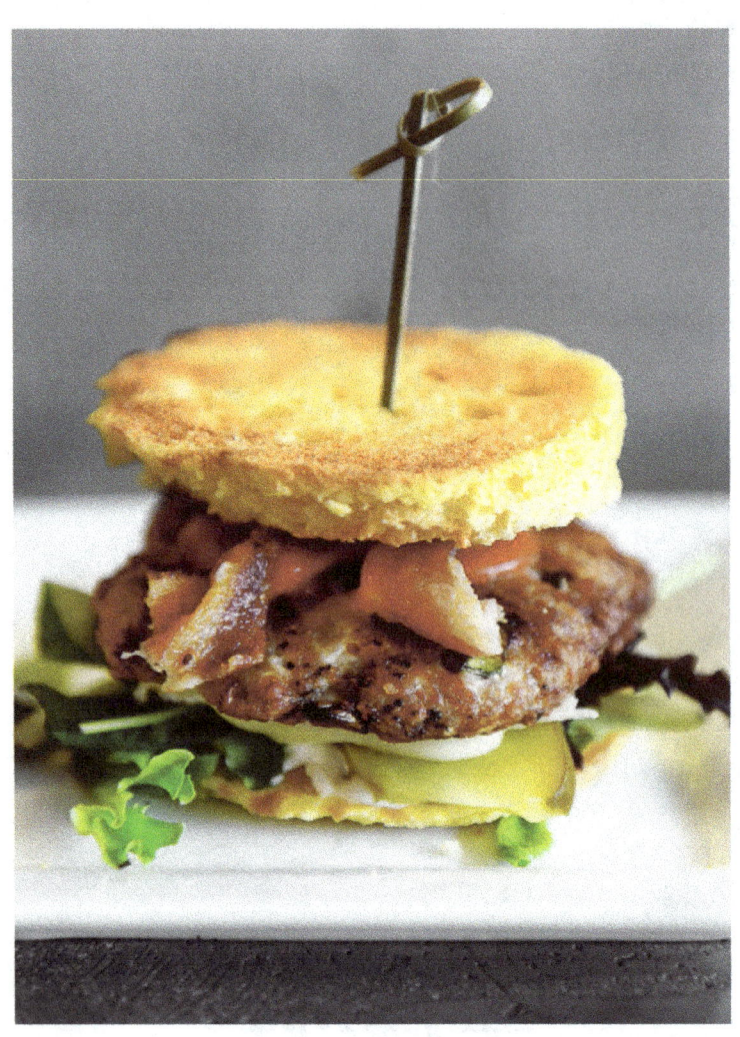

Table of Contents

Introduction

Do you already have these keto must-haves?
Switch to this week-long meal plan and start cooking.

7-Day Keto Meal Plan
This meal plan will make your first week of keto easy as pie. It includes breakfast, lunch, and dinner. Double the portions if you want to make a meal and have leftovers.

MONDAY
Breakfast: Pumpkin Pancakes with Hazelnuts

The flavors of almond flour and pumpkin blend perfectly in these protein-packed pancakes. They're ready in less than half an hour. If you have time, serve them warm with a scoop of Greek yogurt and chopped hazelnuts. One serving will give you almost 400 calories, which can be a good thing if your goal is to have a satisfying breakfast that will keep you full until lunchtime.

Lunch: salmon cakes

You can make these patties a day ahead and heat them up or even eat them cold - they're good either way. With only 283 calories per serving, feel free to have 2-3 servings if you're hungry. They're easy to throw together in a couple of minutes and are perfect served with avocado salsa and sour cream.

Dinner: Keto Roasted Chicken

Nothing beats roast chicken on a lazy weekday. It's simple, delicious, and requires minimal effort. However, you'll have to wait at least 2 hours before you can enjoy this easy dinner. Prepare the chicken a day ahead and once it's done, serve with your favorite keto veggies, cauliflower puree or a different side dish of your liking.

TUESDAY
Breakfast: Frittata Di Cheto

What better way to start the day than with a hearty egg breakfast? This recipe calls for a range of keto-friendly ingredients like bacon, chorizo sausage, avocado, cheddar and cream. The result is a high-fat, low-carb omelet that is both nutritious and satisfying. It's perfect served with your favorite keto bread or a glass of white yogurt.

Lunch: Very chocolate berry protein shake

If you're a fan of uncomplicated lunch, you should definitely try this protein shake. It's made with an almond milk base, frozen berries for added antioxidants, chia seeds for texture and healthy omega-3 fats, and chocolate protein powder for both taste and satiety. With over 130 calories and nearly 14g of protein, you can count on this smoothie to keep you full.

Dinner: Spicy Keto Beef Curry

This is a simple curry recipe that you can make in about an hour. It's made with just a handful of ingredients, but the result is a complex blend of spicy and strong flavors. You can enjoy this meal as is or served with some cauliflower rice.

WEDNESDAY
Breakfast: Keto Raspberry Breakfast Jars.

You can make this simple breakfast the night before to save time. It will be just as good, if not better. Chia seeds combined with creamy coconut milk make a decadent batch. The layer of raspberry and mint will provide your daily dose of vitamin C and powerful antioxidants to help fuel you throughout the day.

Lunch: Keto Falafel Salad

Whether you work from home or outside, this keto falafel salad will satisfy your midday cravings. Keep in mind that it takes at least half an hour and many steps to prepare this meal. We recommend preparing the individual ingredients the night before to save time. Falafel salads are high in fiber and protein, which will reduce hunger at dinner.

Dinner: Corned beef hash and cauliflower

My midweek, most of us are to beat to prepare elaborate dinners. That's where meals like this simple hash come in to save the day. You'll need 30 minutes and 7 ingredients to make this delicious meal. Feel free to have two servings as there are only 123 calories in one serving of this cauliflower. If you want to increase the calorie count even more, add some sour cream.

THURSDAY
Breakfast: Keto Bagel

For a fast and quick breakfast, make these bagels ahead of time and store them in the refrigerator or freezer. Each bagel has almost 130 calories and 7g of protein. Use them to make a keto sandwich with ingredients like ham, cheddar cheese, sliced avocado and scrambled eggs. Alternatively, eat with a buttercream or avocado and serve with your favorite smoothie or Greek yogurt.

Lunch: Italian Keto Rollups

A convenient keto favorite at lunchtime, these rollups take minutes and have all your favorite keto ingredients to boot. Italian cured meats paired with cream cheese and a little chili are all you need to make the base for these rollups. Enjoy on your own for an easy and satisfying snack or with your favorite firecrackers.

Dinner: Beef Keto and Broccoli Stir-Fry

A simple Chinese-style beef and broccoli stir-fry is easy to make when you're too beat up to cook. You'll just need a handful of simple ingredients, 30 minutes of your time, and a deep skillet or wok. Serve it with some cauliflower fried rice to soak up the succulent sauce and get it filling.

FRIDAY
Breakfast: Mini baked omelettes with mushrooms

Another great egg-based breakfast are these mini frittatas. This recipe yields 9 frittatas, each of which provides nearly 140 calories, most coming from fat and protein. Use porcini mushrooms for this recipe or even portobello if that's what you have.

Lunch: Avocado Lime Smoothie

Another great lunchtime smoothie is this green avocado-based smoothie. Almond milk serves as a delicate base here to accentuate the pineapple and lime flavors. The result is a satisfying smoothie drink that is both refreshing and hearty. Seasoned with chia seeds and flavored with a little stevia, this smoothie will keep you on the carb limit and healthy.

Dinner: Roast Beef and Cheese Deli Plate

You can fix this as an appetizer dish or enjoy it as dinner. There's no cooking involved here, simply cutting and arranging the keto-friendly ingredients we know and love. With over 400 calories, 40g of fat and 12g of protein per serving, this dish is definitely satisfying, especially if you eat it with some keto bread.

SATURDAY
Breakfast: Avocado Tuna Salad

To make your Saturday morning special, try this healthy stuffed avocado salad. This recipe yields 2 slices, each providing 222 calories. Packed with anti-inflammatory omega-3 fatty acids from the tuna and heart-healthy monounsaturated fats from the avocados, this avocado dish is a healthy way to start your day.

Lunch: Thai Beef Lettuce Wraps

For fans of Thai flavors, this is the perfect lunchtime meal. Savory beef wrapped in cabbage leaves or romaine lettuce and topped with parsley and mint, this dish is sure to leave you wanting more. This recipe yields a total of 4 servings, each with 370 calories, 14 g of fat, 53 g of protein and only 2 g of net carbs.

Dinner: Spicy Beef Ramen

Ramen is the ultimate comfort food. But it's not really keto-friendly unless you use low-carb noodles like the ones used in this recipe. The dish is made with miracle noodles, which are made with glucomannan, a type of fiber from the konjac plant. In addition to the low-carb noodles, you'll need ground beef, Asian and other spices, and meat broth to make this meal.

SUNDAY
Breakfast Biscuit Sandwiches

Start this Sunday with these filling and tasty sandwiches. The cookies are made with head dough and some herbs for extra flavor. The filling is a simple mix of scrambled eggs, bacon and arugula. You can make the cookie dough and freeze it or store it in the refrigerator. Serve with yogurt, lemon water or a light smoothie.

Lunch: Green Turkey Salad

A simple turkey and vegetable salad can serve as a healthy lunchtime option. This includes cooked, shredded turkey meat, which you can get from leftover turkey or make from scratch using turkey breast. Watercress, arugula, gorgonzola, sliced almonds and balsamic vinegar are just a couple of other ingredients that combine perfectly in this salad.

Dinner: French Onion Soup

And finally, end your first week of keto with a warm bowl of French onion soup - you deserve it! This onion soup is comforting, flavorful, and loaded with keto-friendly ingredients like butter, cheese, and almond flour croutons. It also has over 500 calories, 30g of fat and 50g of protein.

In addition to sticking to these meals, consider adding snacks to your eating plan to hit your daily calories and macros. You can find snack recipes here and here.

Want to know what to expect after your first week of keto?

Well, most people are able to enter ketosis within 3-7 days of starting the keto diet. Signs of ketosis to look out for include:

Ketone breath (a strong fruity smelling breath)
Changes in energy levels
Keto flu (a common side effect of switching to ketosis)
Ketones in urine (measurable with urine strips)
The transition to ketosis is often initially uncomfortable for most people. This is because most are not used to restricting carbohydrates to a level that produces ketosis and their bodies

may react to this change. Another reason you may experience discomfort is because you have developed keto flu, a side effect that includes symptoms such as:

- Headaches
- Muscle pain
- Fatigue
- Palpitations
- Nausea
- Stomachaches
- Foggy brain

These symptoms are most commonly the result of electrolyte imbalances but also changes in blood glucose levels. Fortunately, ketone flu is easy to prevent by staying hydrated, eating enough, and even taking electrolyte supplements. Some people find that ketonic flu is easier to beat by taking MCT oil or exogenous ketones in the first week of a keto diet.

Chapter 1: Keto Appetizers

Bacon-wrapped halloumi cheese

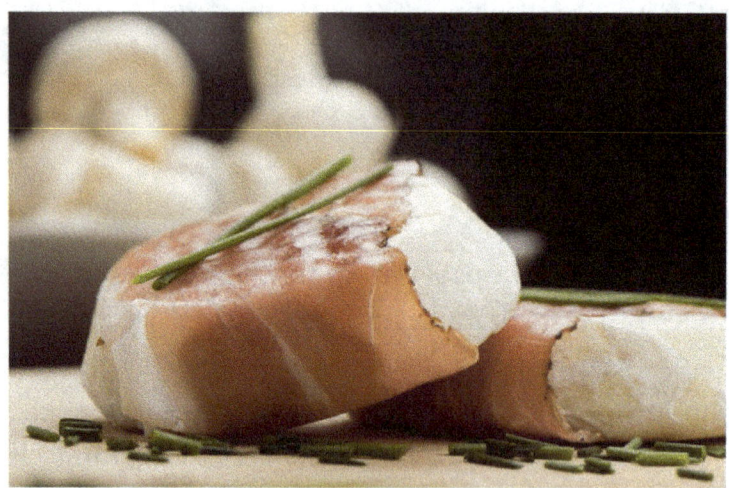

Servings: 2
4g 2% Net carbs
52g 28% Protein
57g 70% Fat
Total: 4 g
(kcal: 748)

Ingredients:
- 8 oz. halloumicheese
- 6 oz. bacon, in slices

Instructions:
1. Preheat the oven to 450°F (225°C).
2. Cutcheeseinto 8–10 pieces.
3. Wrap a piece of bacon around each piece of cheese.
4. Place on a baking sheet and bake in oven until golden brown for 10–15 minutes, flipping halfway through.

Creamy low-carb broccoli and leek soup

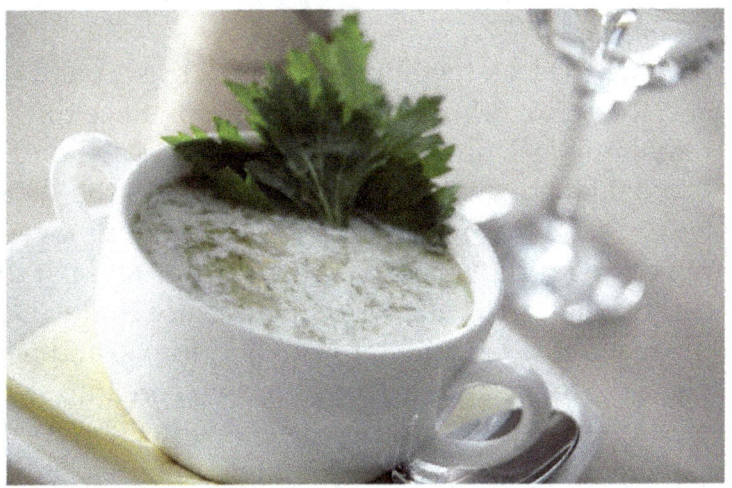

Servings: 4
12g 8% Net carbs
17g 12% Protein
53g 80% Fat
Total: 14 g
(kcal: 590)

Ingredients:
- 1 (3 oz.) leek
- 10 oz. head of broccoli
- 3 cups vegetable stock
- ¼ tsp salt
- 7 oz. (⅘ cup) creamcheese
- 1 cup heavy whippingcream
- ½ tsp ground black pepper
- ½ cup (¾ oz.) freshbasil, chopped
- 1 garlicclove, pressed
- Cheese chips
- 1½ cups (6 oz.) cheddar cheese, or edam cheese, shredded
- ½ tsp paprika powder

15

Instructions:

Broccoli soup
1. Prepare the leek by giving it a quick rinse, pat it dry, and then trim off the rough, green tips. Slice the remaining leek, into thin circles, and discard the root. Next, fill a bowl with cold water and add the sliced leeks. Move them around in the water to remove any remaining dirt or sand, and then strain, and pat dry.
2. Cut off the core of the broccoli and slice thinly. Divide the rest of the broccoli into smaller florets, and reserve.
3. Place the leek and the sliced broccoli core into a medium-size pot. Add the vegetable stock and salt. Cover, and bring to a boil for a few minutes, until the broccoli can be easily pierced with a knife.
4. Lower the heat to medium-low, and add the broccoli florets. Simmer for a few minutes, until the broccoli is bright green and tender. Add the creamcheese, cream, pepper, basil, and garlic.
5. Blend with an immersion blender until desired consistency. If the soup is too thick, thin it out with water. If you'd like it to have a slightly thicker consistency, add a touch of heavy cream.

Cheese chips
1. Preheat oven at 400°F (200°C). Line a large, rimmed baking sheet with parchment paper.
2. Place mounds of the shredded cheese by the tablespoon, 1" (2.5 cm) apart on the parchment paper. Sprinkleeachmound with paprika.
3. Bake on the middle rack, for about 5-6 minutes, or until the cheese has melted. Serve on the side with the broccoli and leek soup.

Keto baked goat cheese with blackberries and roasted pistachios

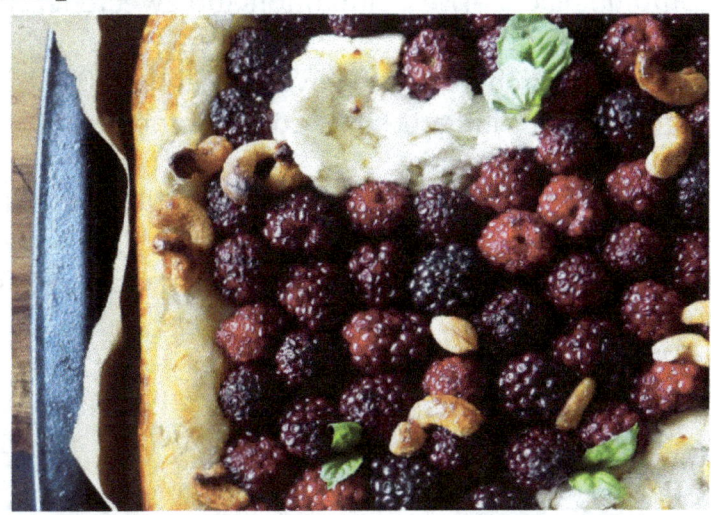

Servings: 4
4g 3% Net carbs
33g 24% Protein
46g 74% Fat
Total: 8 g
(kcal: 584)

Ingredients:
- 1¼ lbs goatcheese
- Blackberry sauce
- 9 oz. freshblackberries
- 1 tbsp erythritol (optional)
- 1 pinch ground cinnamon
- Topping
- 1 oz. pistachio nuts
- salt
- freshrosemary

Instructions:

1. Preheat the oven to 350°F (180°C).
2. Combine blackberries, cinnamon and sweetener, if using. Set aside.
3. Bake the goat cheese in the oven for about 10 to 12 minutes or until it gets some color. Remove and letsit for a few minutes.
4. Roughly chop the pistachios and roast them in a dry frying pan. Season with salt.
5. Top the goat cheese with blackberry, roasted pistachio and rosemary.

Low-carb beef empanadas with dip

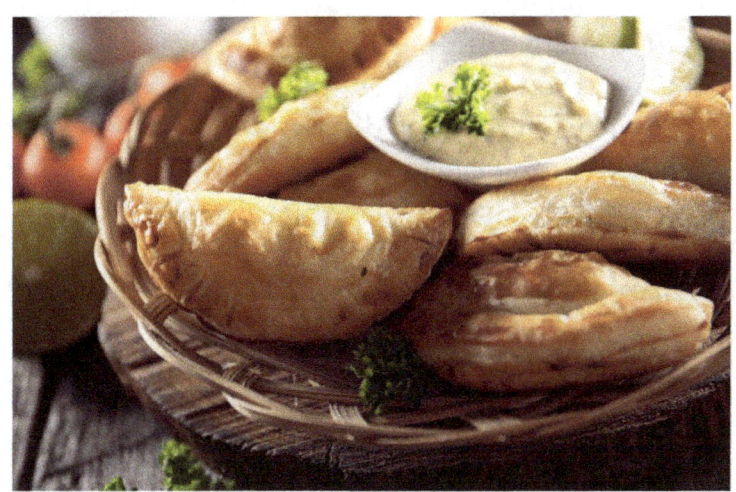

Servings: 4
7g 6% Net carbs
19g 14% Protein
48g 81% Fat
Total: 9 g
(kcal: 554)

Ingredients:

Empanada dough
- 1¼ cups (5 oz.) almondflour
- 1 tsp bakingpowder
- ½ tsp cream of tartar
- 1 tsp xanthangum
- 2 eggs, divided
- 2 tbsp butter, at room temperature
- 2 tbsp ricotta cheese
- 1 tsp heavy whipping cream (for egg wash)

Filling
- 3 tbsp olive oil
- ¼ (1 oz.) red onion, finelychopped

- 1 garlicclove, minced
- ¼ lb ground beef
- ¼ cup tomato sauce
- ¼ (1¼ oz.) red bellpepper, minced
- 1 (7 oz.) zucchini, finelydiced
- 1 tsp salt, or to taste
- ½ tsp pepper
- 1 egg, hard boiled and finely chopped

Dippingsauce
- ½ cup sourcream
- ½ tsp garlicpowder
- ½ tsp salt
- 1 freshjalapeño, chopped
- 1/3 oz. (9 tbsp) freshcilantro

Instructions:

For the filling
1. Heat the oil over medium heat. Stir in the onion and cook while stirring until it turns translucent.
2. Add in the garlic and ground beef, stirring until meat browns.
3. Pour in the tomato sauce, add bell pepper, zucchini, salt, and pepper. Stir and cover. Simmer for 3 minutes.
4. Taste and season with salt and pepper to taste if needed. Remove from the heat. Mix in the minced egg and set aside.

Empanadas
5. In a mixing bowl, whisk to combine almond flour, baking powder, cream of tartar, and xanthan gum.
6. Add the butter, ricotta, and half of the eggs.
7. Using the hook attachment of a mixer, knead until it has become a smooth ball of dough (about 2 minutes).
8. Remove from the mixer, wrap in plastic film and let it rest in the refrigerator for an hour.

9. Cut parchment paper into squares, roughly 7" x 7" (18 x 18 cm).
10. Once the dough is chilled, remove it from the refrigerator, cut them into pieces, and form each piece into a ball.
11. Press each ball between two pieces of parchment paper using a cutting board (or extend using a rolling pin) to make a flat disc that is 5" (13 cm) in diameter.
12. Peel off the top layer of paper and reuse for the other balls, leaving the discs on the bottom paper. The dough is softer and more delicate than the traditional empanadas dough, so you have to handle it with a bit more care. Set the discs aside.
13. Split the remaining egg into yolk and white. Set the white aside. Whisk the yolk and heavy cream together. Set itasidetoo.

Baked mini bell peppers

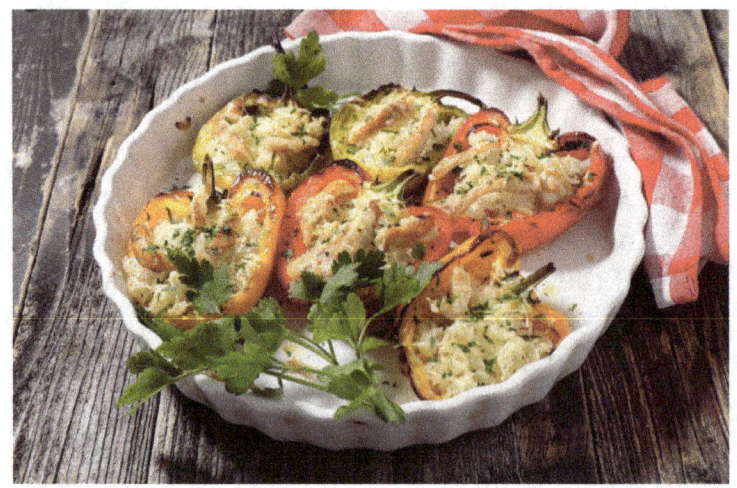

Servings: 4
7g 7% Net carbs
12g 11% Protein
38g 82% Fat
Total: 8 g
(kcal: 411)

Ingredients:
- 8 oz. mini bell peppers, about 2 per serving
- 1 oz. air-dried chorizo, finely chopped
- 1 tbsp fresh thyme, finely chopped or fresh cilantro
- 8 oz. (1 cup) creamcheese
- ½ tbsp mildchipotle paste
- 2 tbsp olive oil
- 1 cup (4 oz.) shredded cheddar cheese

Instructions:
1. Set the oven to 325°F (200°C). Split the bell peppers lengthwise and remove the core.
2. Finely chop the chorizo and the herbs.
3. Mix together the cream cheese, spices and oil in a small bowl. Add the chorizo and herbs. Stiruntilsmooth.
4. Fill the bell peppers with the mixture and place in a greased baking dish.
5. Sprinkle shredded cheese on top. Bake in the oven for 15–20 minutes or until the cheese is melted and golden brown.

Keto wraps with avocado and shrimp salad

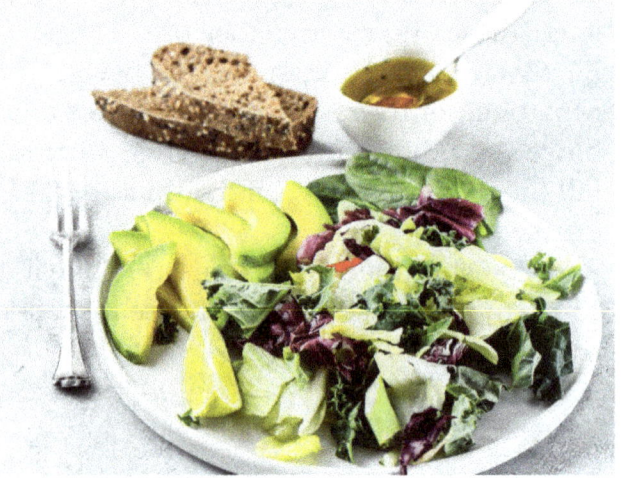

Servings: 2
6g3%Net carbs
27g14%Protein
71g83%Fat
Total: 20 g
(kcal: 802)

Ingredients:

Shrimp salad
- 2 (14 oz.) avocados
- 1 tsp lime juice
- 6 oz. shrimp, cooked and peeled
- 1 (1½ oz.) celerystalk
- 1 tsp sambal oelek or chili paste
- ¼ cup mayonnaise or vegan mayonnaise
- ¼ cup (1/8 oz.) fresh cilantro or fresh parsley

Wraps
- 4 eggs
- 1 oz. butter or coconut oil
- salt and pepper

Instructions:

Wraps
1. Whisk the eggs with a pinch of salt and pepper.
2. Bring out a medium-sized frying pan and let the butter melt slowly over medium-low heat.
3. Add half of the batter and cook until the wrap has firmed up. Flip if you want, but this is not really necessary. The wraps are not supposed to turn color, just get firm.
4. Repeat with remaining batter.

Salad
5. Split and scoop out the avocado. Dice the avocado into ½-inch cubes and place in a bowl, squeeze lime juice over them and stir.
6. Slice the celery thinly. Add to the bowl with the avocado.
7. Add mayonnaise, sambal oelek, and finely chopped cilantro.
8. Mix well and stir in the cooked shrimp carefully. Salt and pepper to taste.

Keto butter chicken wings

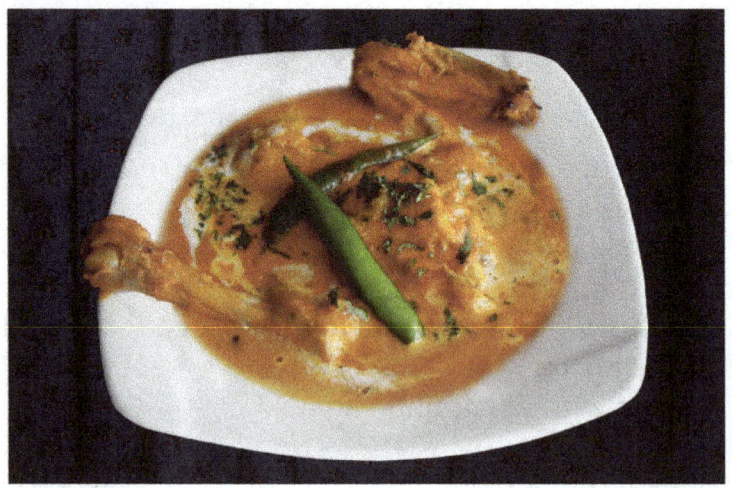

Servings: 4
6g 3% Net carbs
46g 26% Protein
54g 70% Fat
Total: 7 g
(kcal: 704)

Ingredients:

Chatpatadip
- ¾ cup Greek yogurt
- 2 tbsp creamcheese
- ¼ tsp garlicpowder
- ¼ tsp chaatmasala
- 1 tbsp finelychopped, freshcilantro
- salt

Chicken wings
- 2 lbs chicken wings
- 1 tsp salt
- 1 tsp tandooriseasoning
- 1 tbsp ghee

Buttersauce
- 2 oz. butter
- 1 tsp ginger garlic paste
- ½ tsp chili powder
- ½ tsp turmeric
- ½ tsp coriander, ground
- ½ tsp garammasalaseasoning
- ½ tsp ground cumin
- ½ cup tomato puree
- ¼ cup water
- 1 tsp dried fenugreek (kasoorimethi)
- 1 tsp salt
- freshcilantro, chopped, for serving
- ¼ cup heavy whippingcream
- 2 tbsp finelychopped freshcilantro

Instructions:

Chatpatadip
1. In a medium-sized bowl, mix together the yogurt, cream cheese, garlic powder, chaat masala, and cilantro. Season with salt, to taste.
2. Cover and refrigerate for 30 minutes or more, until serving.

Chicken wings
3. Preheat oven to 400°F (200°C). Set aside a rimmed baking sheet with a fitted rack, lined with parchment paper.
4. In a large bowl, whisk together the salt, tandoori masala, and ghee. Add the chicken wings, and toss them together to completely coat.
5. Using tongs, place wings on the baking tray rack, and bake for 25 minutes. Transfer wings into a large bowl and set aside. Meanwhile, prepare the butter sauce.

Buttersauce

6. Heat the butter, ginger garlic paste, chili powder, turmeric, ground coriander, garam masala, and cumin in a small saucepan, over low heat. Whisktogetheruntilbutterismelted and combined.
7. Add the tomato purée, water, and fenugreek. Stir together, cover, and cook for 5 minutes.
8. Stir in the salt, and cook for another 5 minutes. Add the cilantro and cream, whisk together, and cook uncovered for a few minutes, until the sauce thickens. Remove from heat.
9. Pour 3/4 sauce over the wings, and toss to coat. Using tongs or a slotted spoon, return wings to the baking rack and bake for 10 minutes, or longer for desired crispiness (reserve the leftover butter sauce in the bowl).
10. Transfer baked wings into the bowl containing the 1/4 reserved butter sauce, and toss to coat.
11. Sprinkle extra cilantro over the wings, and serve with the chatpata dip on the side.

Keto pimiento cheese meatballs

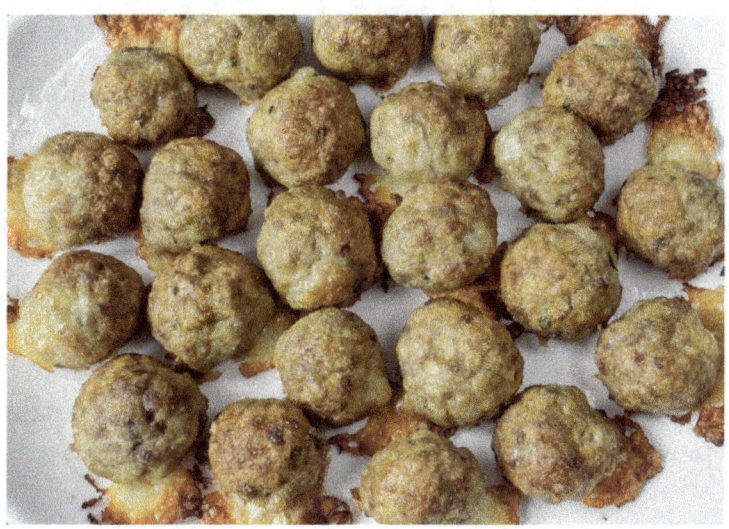

Servings: 4
1g 1% Net carbs
41g 26% Protein
52g 73% Fat
Total: 2 g
(kcal: 648)

Ingredients:

Pimiento cheese
- 1/3 cup mayonnaise or vegan mayonnaise
- ¼ cup pimientos or pickled jalapeños
- 1 tsp paprika powder or chili powder
- 1 tbsp Dijonmustard
- 1 pinch cayenne pepper
- 1 cup (4 oz.) grated cheddar cheese

Meatballs
- 1½ lbs ground beef or ground turkey
- 1 egg
- salt and pepper

- 2 tbsp butter, for frying

Instructions:
1. Start by mixing all ingredients for the pimiento cheese in a large bowl.
2. Add ground beef and the egg to the cheese mixture. Use a wooden spoon or clean hands to combine. Salt and pepper to taste.
3. Form large meatballs and fry them in butter or oil in a skillet on medium heat until they are thoroughly cooked.
4. Serve with a side dish of your choice, a green salad and perhaps a homemade mayonnaise.

Spicy keto deviled eggs

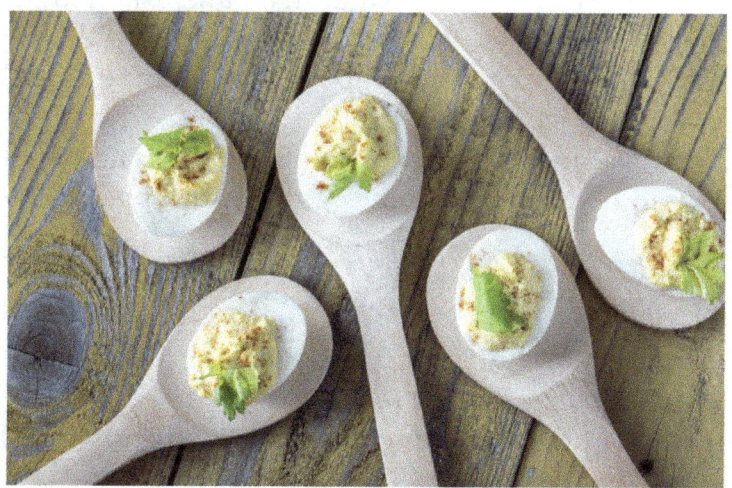

Servings: 6
1g 2% Net carbs
6g 12% Protein
18g 86% Fat
Total: 1 g
(kcal: 197)

Ingredients:

- 6 eggs
- 1 tbsp red curry paste
- ½ cup mayonnaise or vegan mayonnaise
- ¼ tsp salt
- ½ tbsp poppyseeds

Instructions:

1. Place the eggs in cold water in a pan, just enough water to cover the eggs. Bring to a boilwithout a lid.
2. Let the eggs simmer for about eight minutes. Cool quickly in ice-cold water.
3. Remove the egg shells. Cut off both ends and split the egg in half. Scoop out the egg yolk and place in a small bowl.
4. Place the egg whites on a plate and let sit in the refrigerator.
5. Mix curry paste, mayonnaise and egg yolks into a smooth batter. Salt to taste.
6. Bring out the egg whites from the refrigerator and apply the batter.
7. Sprinkle the seeds on top and serve.

Keto mozzarella-stuffed meatballs

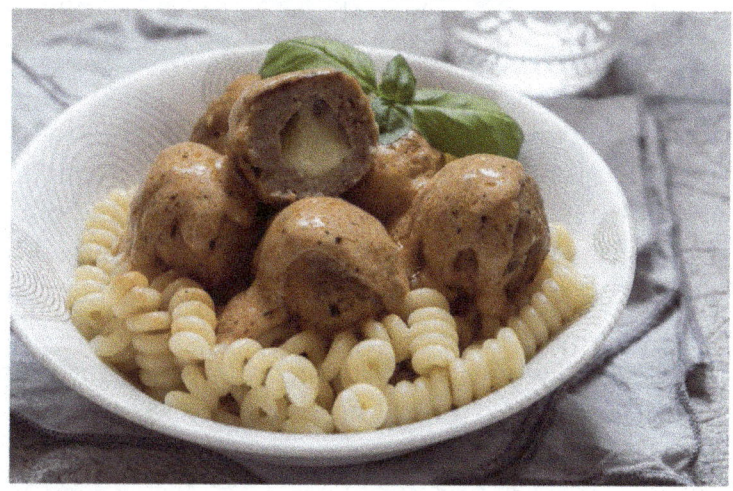

Servings: 4
2g 1% Net carbs
40g 32% Protein
36g 66% Fat
Total: 2 g
(kcal: 501)

Ingredients:

- 1½ lbs ground beef or ground turkey
- 2 tbsp heavy whippingcream
- 2 garliccloves, minced
- 1 tbsp driedbasil
- 1 tsp salt
- ¼ tsp ground black pepper
- 4 oz. (1 cup) shredded mozzarella cheese
- 2 tbsp butter, for frying

Instructions:

1. In a large bowl, combine the ground meat with cream, garlic, basil, salt, and ground black pepper. Mix well with your hands or a large wooden fork.
2. Form the balls using wet hands. The bigger you make them the longer they will take to cook. Flatten them out in your hand and place a pile of cheese in the middle of the patty. Wrap the meat around the cheese and form it into a ball. Repeat until you've used all of the meat and cheese.
3. In a large frying pan, fry the meatballs in butter on medium-high heat until nicely browned.

Scallops parmesan

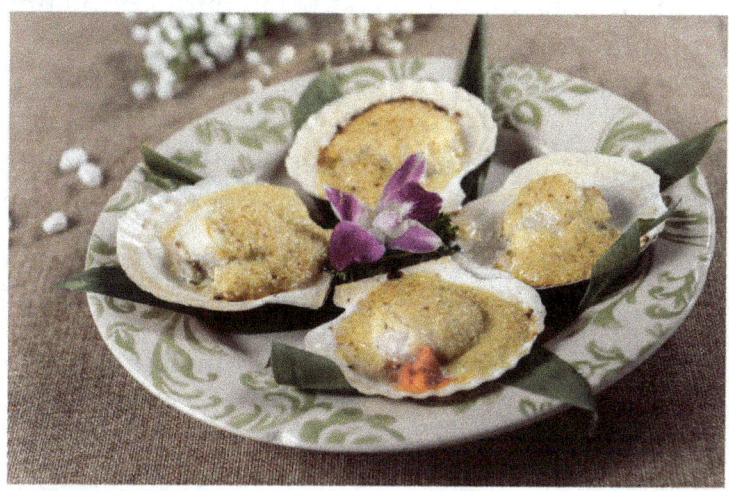

Servings: 4
5g 7% Net carbs
13g 16% Protein
27g 77% Fat
Total: 6 g
(kcal: 325)

Ingredients:
- 8 scallops
- 1 tbsp butter
- 1 (1 oz.) shallot, finelychopped
- ¼ cup white wine
- 1 cup heavy whippingcream
- ¼ cup gratedparmesancheese
- salt and pepper

Instructions:

1. Chop the shallot finely and fry in butter or oil until soft without letting it turn brown.
2. Add wine and stir. Let simmer until most of the wine is gone.
3. Pour in the cream and let boil together for a while.
4. Stir in parmesan cheese. Salt and pepper. Remove from heat.
5. Brown the scallops for no more than 30 seconds on each side, in a hot pan until nicely browned.
6. Bake in the oven, using the broil function for a few minutes at 450°F (225°C), or until the sauce has turned golden brown.

Hot keto shrimp cocktail

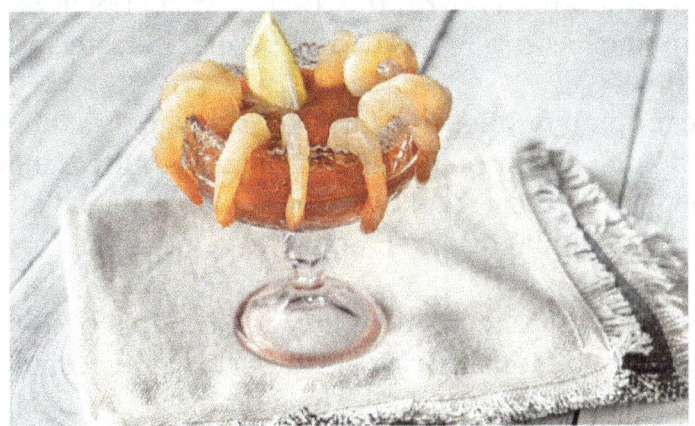

Servings: 4
2g 2% Net carbs
12g 10% Protein
49g 88% Fat
Total: 3 g
(kcal: 503)

Ingredients:
- 2 tbsp coconut oil or ghee
- 1 garlicclove
- 12 oz. peeledshrimp
- ½ tsp chili flakes
- 2 tbsp finelychoppedfreshparsley
- salt and pepper

Thousandislanddip
- 1 cup mayonnaise
- ½ tbsp tomato paste
- ½ tbsp lemonjuice
- 1 tsp hot sauce
- 1 tsp paprika powder
- 1 tsp onionpowder
- salt and pepper

Instructions:

1. Add all ingredients for the dip to a small bowl. Stir to combine. Season with salt and pepper to taste and set aside.
2. Heat up oil or ghee in a large frying pan. Use the side of a knife or a spoon to smash the garlic cloves, but keep them (mostly) in one piece. Add smashed cloves to the oil to flavor it; remember to remove the cloves before serving.
3. Add shrimp to the pan and fry for a couple of minutes on each side if using raw shrimp. They are done as soon as they have turned a nice pink color. If using pre-cooked shrimp, just heat them up quickly in the pan and allow them to get flavor from oil and garlic.
4. Add chili flakes, salt, and pepper to taste. Chop the parsley finely and sprinkle on top.
5. Fried shrimp are best served right away with a side of creamy sauce for dipping.

Keto stuffed mushrooms

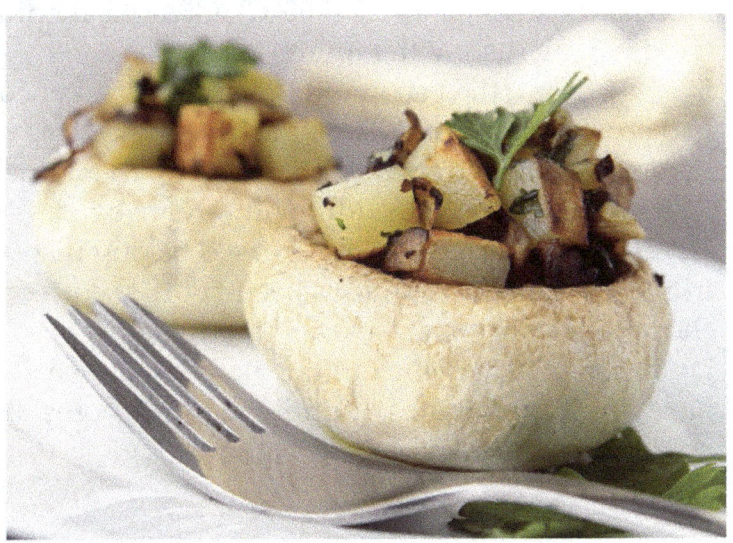

Servings: 4
6g 4% Net carbs
25g 18% Protein
48g 78% Fat
Total: 7 g
(kcal: 555)

Ingredients:
- 8 oz. bacon
- 12 mushrooms
- 2 tbsp butter
- 9 oz. (1¼ cups) creamcheese
- 3 tbsp freshchives, finelychopped
- 1 tsp paprika powder
- salt and pepper

Instructions:

1. Preheat the oven to 400°F (200°C). Grease a medium-sized baking dish with butter.
2. Start by frying the bacon until really crispy. Let cool and crush into crumbs. Save the bacon fat.
3. Remove the mushroom stems and chop them finely. Sauté in the bacon fat, adding butter if needed.
4. Place the mushrooms in the greased baking dish.
5. In a bowl, mix the crumbled bacon with the fried, chopped mushroom stems and the remaining ingredients. Add some of the mix to eachmushroom.
6. Bake for 25-30 minutes or until the mushrooms turn golden brown.

Keto oven-baked Brie cheese

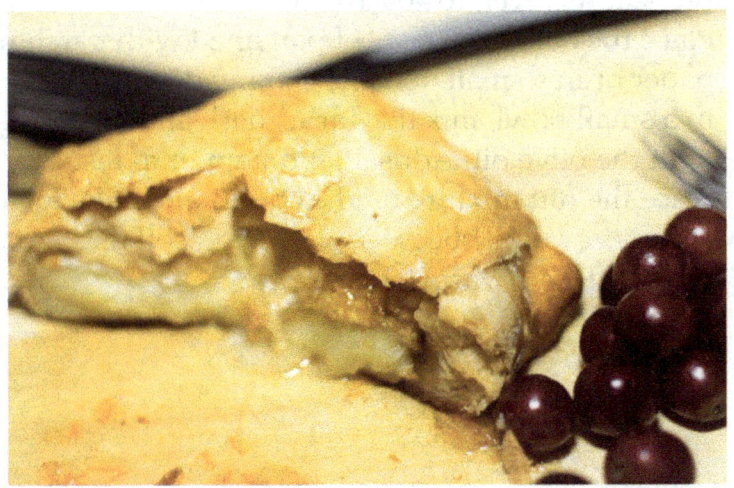

Servings: 4
1g 1% Net carbs
15g 17% Protein
31g 82% Fat
Total: 3 g
(kcal: 341)

Ingredients:
- 9 oz. Brie cheese or Camembert cheese
- 1 garlicclove, minced
- 1 tbsp freshrosemary, coarselychopped
- 2 oz. pecans or walnuts, coarsely chopped
- 1 tbsp olive oil
- salt and pepper

Instructions:
1. Preheat the oven to 400°F (200°C).
2. Place the cheese on a sheet pan lined with parchment paper or in a small nonstick baking dish.
3. In a small bowl, mix the garlic, herb and nuts together with the olive oil. Addsalt and pepper to taste.
4. Place the nut mixture on the cheese and bake for 10 minutes or until cheese is warm and soft and nuts are toasted. Serve warm or lukewarm.

Keto salmon-filled avocados

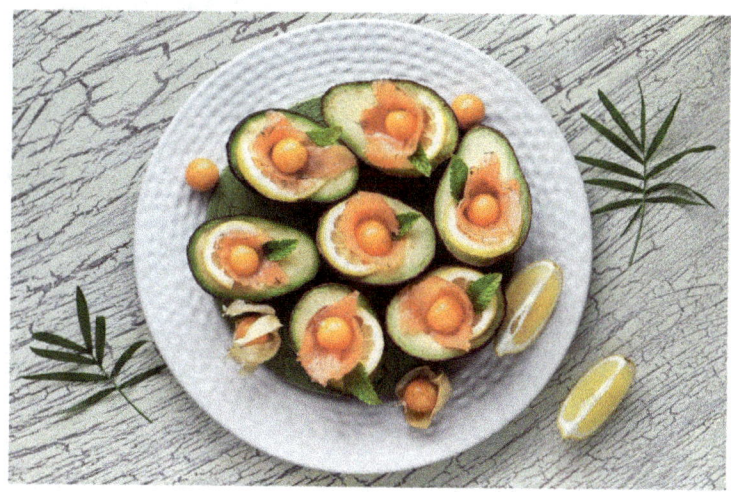

Servings: 2
6g 5% Net carbs
26g 19% Protein
45g 76% Fat
Total: 20 g
(kcal: 567)

Ingredients:
- 2 (14 oz.) avocados
- 8 oz. smokedsalmon
- ½ cup sourcream
- salt and pepper
- 2 tbsp lemonjuice (optional)

Instructions:
1. Cut avocados in half and remove the pit.
2. Place a dollop of crème fraiche or mayonnaise in the hollow of the avocado and add smoked salmon on top.
3. Season to taste with salt and a squeeze lemon juice for extra flavor (and to keep the avocado from turning brown).

Keto cauliflower soup with crispy pancetta

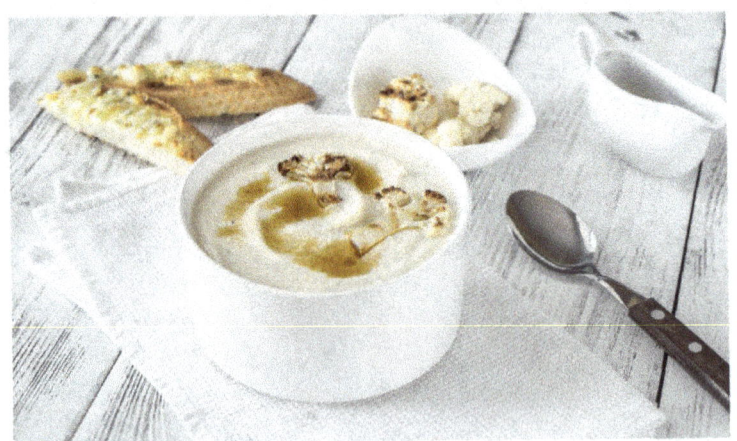

Servings: 6
6g 4% Net carbs
11g 8% Protein
52g 88% Fat
Total: 9 g
(kcal: 527)

Ingredients:
- 1 lb cauliflower, cut into small florets, divided
- 1 tbsp butter
- 7 oz. pancetta, diced or bacon
- 3 oz. pecans, coarselychopped
- 1 tsp paprika powder or smoked chili powder
- 4 cups chicken broth or vegetable stock
- 7 oz. (4/5 cup) creamcheese
- 1 tbsp Dijonmustard
- 4 oz. (½ cup) unsaltedbutter
- ¾ tsp salt
- ½ tsp pepper

Instructions:

1. Chop a handful of the cauliflower florets, into ¼ inch (0.5 cm) pieces.
2. Melt the butter in a medium-sized frying pan, over medium-high heat. Add the chopped cauliflower pieces, and pancetta. Sauté for about 8-10 minutes or until the pancetta becomes crispy. During the last few minutes, stir in the pecans and paprika. Set aside.
3. Add the broth and the rest of the cauliflower florets to a medium-sized, soup pot. Cover and bring to a boil for a couple of minutes, over high heat.
4. Reduce the temperature to medium, and add the cream cheese, mustard, butter, salt, and pepper. Using an immersion blender, combine the ingredients to the desired consistency; blending the mixture for a longer time will produce a creamier soup.
5. To serve, ladle the soup into bowls, and top with the pancetta-pecan mixture.

Keto tortilla pizza

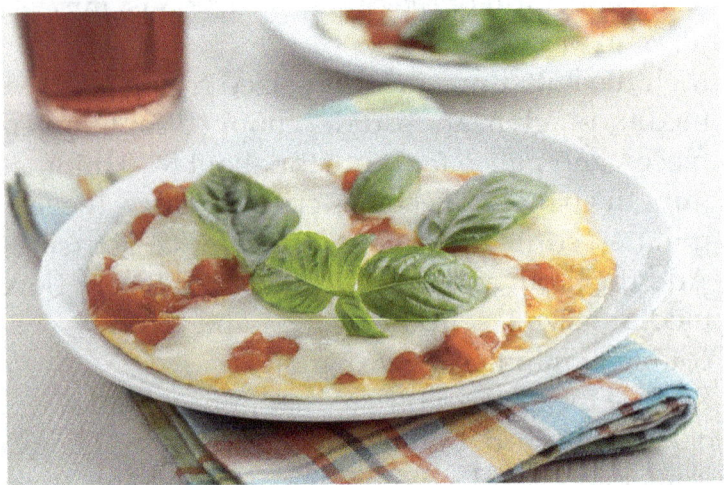

Servings: 4
5g 6% Net carbs
21g 22% Protein
30g 72% Fat
Total: 6 g
(kcal: 377)

Ingredients:

Low-carb tortillas
- 2 large eggs
- 2 large, eggwhites
- 6 oz. (¾ cup) cream cheese, at room temperature
- ¼ tsp salt
- 1 tsp ground psylliumhuskpowder
- 1 tbsp coconutflour

Topping
- ½ cup unsweetened tomato sauce, divided
- 2 cups (8 oz.) shredded, mozzarella cheese
- 2 tsp dried basil or dried oregano

Instructions:

Tortillas

1. Preheat the oven to 400°F (200°C). Set aside (2) baking sheets, lined with parchment paper.
2. Add the eggs and egg whites to a large mixing bowl. Using an electric mixer, whisk together for a few minutes until fluffy. Add the cream cheese, and whisk together until it becomes a smooth batter.
3. In a small bowl, mix together the salt, psyllium husk, and coconut flour. Add one spoonful of this mixture into the batter, whisk together, and repeat until combined. Let the batter sit for a few minutes, or until the batter has thickened (see tip).
4. Use a spatula to spread the batter on the baking sheets, into 4-6 thin circles, or 2 thin rectangles (no more than ¼" or 5 mm thick).
5. Bake on the middle and upper racks for about 15 minutes, or until the edges are lightly browned. Remove from oven, and set aside.

Pizza

6. Increase the oven temperature to 450°F (225°C).
7. Spread the tomato sauce onto each crust, top with the cheese, basil, or oregano, and return to middle and upper oven racks.
8. Bake for about 5 minutes, or until the cheese is melted and golden. Set aside to cool for a few minutes, and then slice, and serve.

Goat cheese salad with balsamico butter

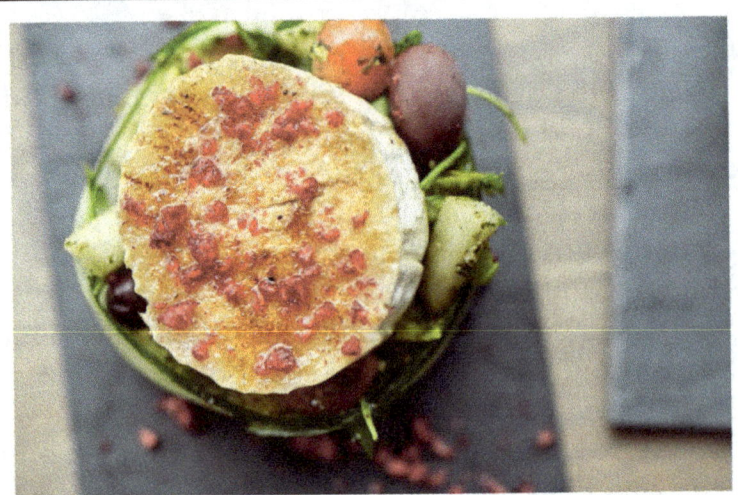

Servings: 2
3g 1% Net carbs
37g 18% Protein
73g 80% Fat
Total: 5 g
(kcal: 826)

Ingredients:

- 10 oz. goatcheese
- ¼ cup (1¼ oz.) pumpkinseeds
- 2 oz. butter
- 1 tbsp balsamicvinegar
- 3 oz. (2¾ cups) baby spinach

Instructions:
1. Preheat the oven to 400°F (200°C).
2. Put slices of goat cheese in a greased baking dish and bake in the oven for 10 minutes.
3. While the goat cheese is in the oven, toast pumpkin seeds in a dry frying pan over fairly high temperature until they get some color and start to pop.
4. Lower the heat, add butter and let simmer until it turns a golden brown color and a pleasant nutty scent. Add balsamic vinegar and let boil for a few more minutes. Turn off the heat.
5. Spread out baby spinach on a plate. Place the cheese on top and add the balsamico butter.

Buttery harissa shrimp skewers

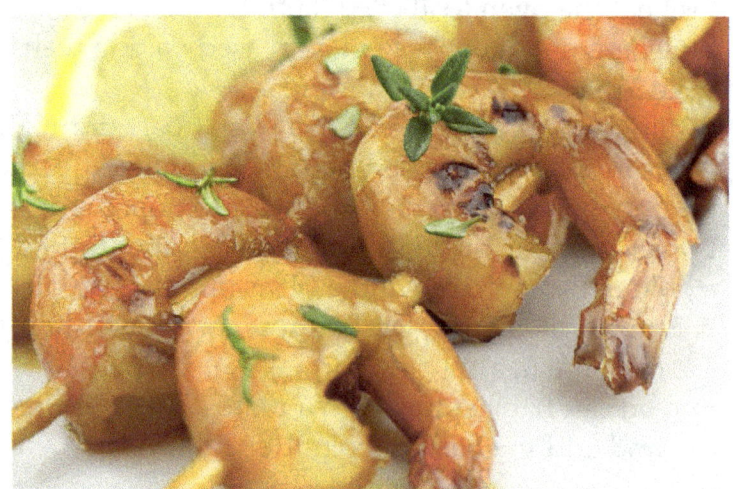

Servings: 4
2g 6% Net carbs
16g 38% Protein
10g 56% Fat
Total: 3 g

Ingredients:
- 1 lb large shrimp, peeled and deveined
- sea salt and ground black pepper
- 3 tbsp butter, melted
- 2 tbsp harissa paste
- 1 tbsp fresh lime juice
- ½ tsp seasalt
- 2 garliccloves, minced
- 1 lime in wedges, for serving
- 4 skewers (metal or wooden)

Instructions:
1. Season the shrimp generously with salt and pepper and set aside.
2. To a large mixing bowl, add the butter, harissa, lime juice, salt, and garlic. Whisk to combine.
3. Add the shrimp to the mixing bowl and toss to coat in the sauce. Letmarinade for 60 minutes.
4. Thread the shrimp onto the skewers and pour any remaining marinade over top.
5. Heat a large grill pan over medium high heat. Once the pan is hot, add the skewers to the pan and cook, rotating halfway through, until the shrimp are cooked all the way through, about 5 minutes.
6. Serve with lime wedges.

Keto taco shells

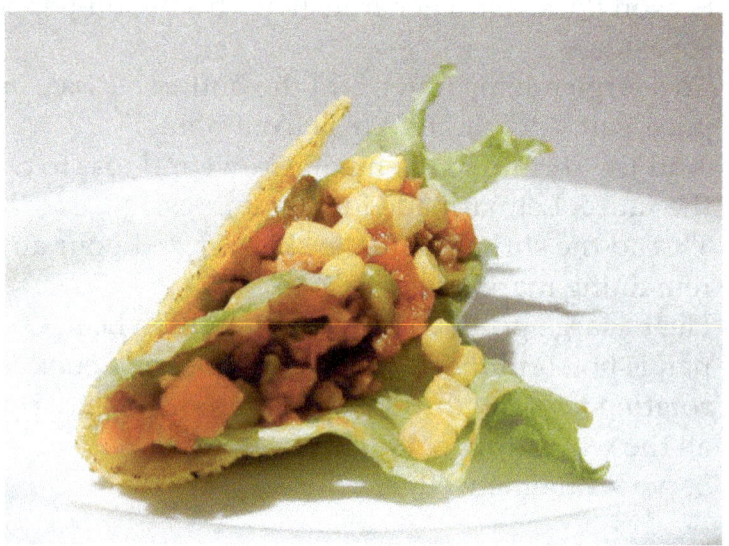

Servings: 4
2g 3% Net carbs
13g 23% Protein
19g 74% Fat
Total: 2 g
(kcal: 228)

Ingredients:
- 2 cups (8 oz.) shredded cheddar cheese
- ½ tsp ground cumin

Instructions:
1. Preheat the oven to 400°F (200°C). Mix cheese and cumin. Form six or eight piles of the cheese on a baking sheet lined with parchment paper. Leave plenty of room in between piles, or the cheese might melt together.
2. Bake in the oven for 10–15 minutes or until the cheese is bubbling with golden brown patches — burned cheese doesn't taste good so watch carefully. Let cool for 30 seconds.
3. Place a rack over the sink.
4. Carefully, place the cheese "tortillas" on the rack. Before the cheese completely cools, allow the edges of each round to drape down between the bars of the rack, forming the taco shell shape.
5. Let cool completely. Serve with fillings of your choice.

Keto bread twists

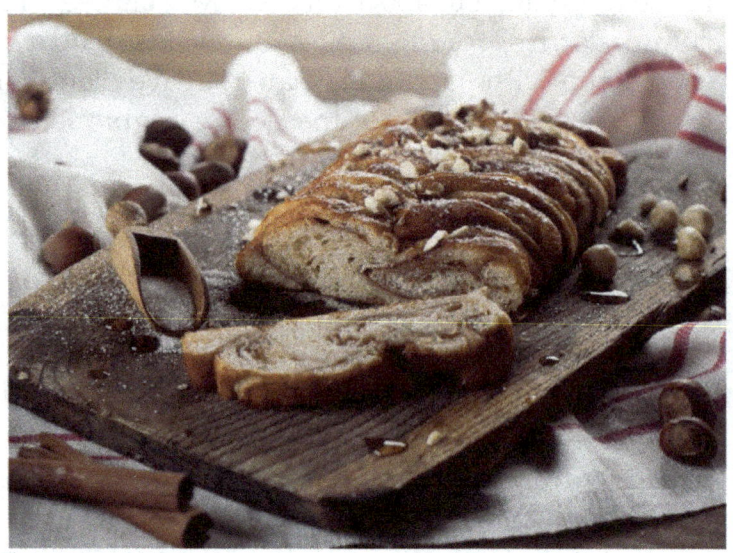

Servings: 10
1g 3% Net carbs
7g 16% Protein
16g 81% Fat
Total: 1 g
(kcal: 181)

Ingredients:

- ½ cup (2 oz.) almondflour
- ¼ cup (¾ oz.) coconutflour
- ½ tsp salt
- 1 tsp bakingpowder
- 1 egg, beaten
- 2 oz. butter
- 12⁄3 cups (6½ oz.) shredded mozzarella cheese
- ¼ cup (2 oz.) green pesto
- 1 egg, beaten, for brushing the top

Instructions:

1. Preheat the oven to 350°F (175°C).
2. Mix all dry ingredients in a bowl. Add the egg and combine.
3. Melt the butter and the cheese together in a pot on low heat. Stir until the batter is smooth.
4. Slowly add the butter-cheese batter to the dry mixture bowl and mix together into a firm dough.
5. Place the dough on parchment paper that is the size of a rectangular cookie sheet. Use a rolling pin and make a rectangle, about 1/5-inch (5 mm) thick.
6. Spread pesto on top and cut into 1-inch (2.5 cm) strips. Twist them and place on a baking sheet lined with parchment paper. Brush twists with the whiskedegg.
7. Bake in the oven for 15–20 minutes until they're golden brown.

Keto butter chicken wings

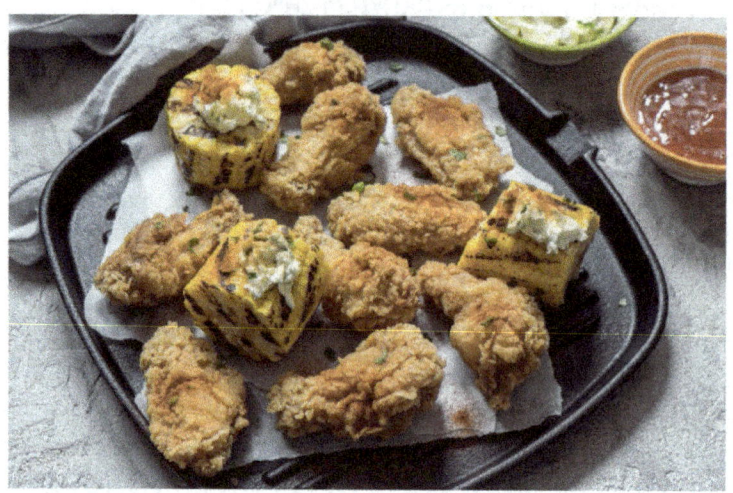

Servings: 4
6g 3% Net carbs
46g 26% Protein
54g 70% Fat
Total: 7 g
(kcal: 704)

Ingredients:

Chatpatadip
- ¾ cup Greek yogurt
- 2 tbsp creamcheese
- ¼ tsp garlicpowder
- ¼ tsp chaatmasala
- 1 tbsp finelychopped, freshcilantro
- salt

Chicken wings
- 2 lbs chicken wings
- 1 tsp salt
- 1 tsp tandooriseasoning
- 1 tbsp ghee

Buttersauce
- 2 oz. butter
- 1 tsp ginger garlic paste
- ½ tsp chili powder
- ½ tsp turmeric
- ½ tsp coriander, ground
- ½ tsp garammasalaseasoning
- ½ tsp ground cumin
- ½ cup tomato puree
- ¼ cup water
- 1 tsp dried fenugreek (kasoorimethi)
- 1 tsp salt
- freshcilantro, chopped, for serving
- ¼ cup heavy whippingcream
- 2 tbsp finelychopped freshcilantro

Instructions:

Chatpatadip
1. In a medium-sized bowl, mix together the yogurt, cream cheese, garlic powder, chaat masala, and cilantro. Season with salt, to taste.
2. Cover and refrigerate for 30 minutes or more, until serving.

Chicken wings
3. Preheat oven to 400°F (200°C). Set aside a rimmed baking sheet with a fitted rack, lined with parchment paper.
4. In a large bowl, whisk together the salt, tandoori masala, and ghee. Add the chicken wings, and toss them together to completely coat.
5. Using tongs, place wings on the baking tray rack, and bake for 25 minutes. Transfer wings into a large bowl and set aside. Meanwhile, prepare the butter sauce.

Buttersauce

6. Heat the butter, ginger garlic paste, chili powder, turmeric, ground coriander, garam masala, and cumin in a small saucepan, over low heat. Whisktogetheruntilbutterismelted and combined.
7. Add the tomato purée, water, and fenugreek. Stir together, cover, and cook for 5 minutes.
8. Stir in the salt, and cook for another 5 minutes. Add the cilantro and cream, whisk together, and cook uncovered for a few minutes, until the sauce thickens. Remove from heat.
9. Pour 3/4 sauce over the wings, and toss to coat. Using tongs or a slotted spoon, return wings to the baking rack and bake for 10 minutes, or longer for desired crispiness (reserve the leftover butter sauce in the bowl).
10. Transfer baked wings into the bowl containing the 1/4 reserved butter sauce, and toss to coat.
11. Sprinkle extra cilantro over the wings, and serve with the chatpata dip on the side.

Keto chicken liver paté with thyme butter

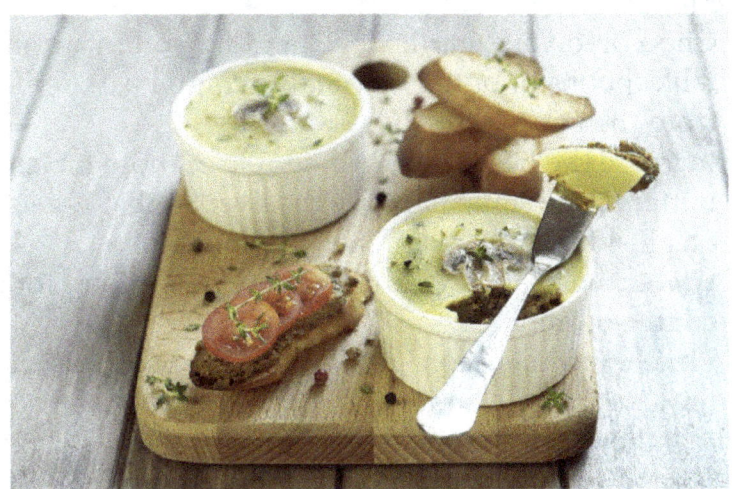

Servings: 10
2g 2% Net carbs
8g 11% Protein
30g 87% Fat
Total: 2 g
(kcal: 305)

Ingredients

Chicken liver paté
- 1 (4 oz.) red onion
- 1 garlicclove
- 8 oz. butter
- 2 tbsp brandy or port wine or other type of liquor that you like (optional)
- 1 tbsp tomato paste
- 1 lb chicken livers

Thymebutter
- 4 oz. butter
- 1 tbsp driedthyme
- 1 tsp ground black pepper

Instructions:
1. Chop onion and garlic finely and fry soft in a couple of tablespoons of butter on medium high heat. Remove from the pan.
2. Increase the heat and add a couple of more tablespoons butter to the same pan. Fry the liver so that it gets fried on all sides. Add liquor. Salt and pepper.
3. Lower the heat and reduce the juices. Let cool for a couple of minutes.
4. Place the fried onion, garlic and liver in a food processor or a blender and mix into a smooth batter together with the rest of the butter and tomato paste. Spread out in a small baking dish, about 7 x 8 inches (18 x 20 cm).
5. Add four ounces of butter for the topping to a small pan and melt carefully on medium heat. Let the white milk protein sink to the bottom and carefully pour the cleared butter into a small bowl.
6. Stir in thyme and pepper. Pour the melted butter over the paté batter and let cool in the refrigerator.
7. Serve on seed crackers or thin slices of low-carb bread with pickled red onions or cucumbers.

Chicken wings with blue cheese dressing

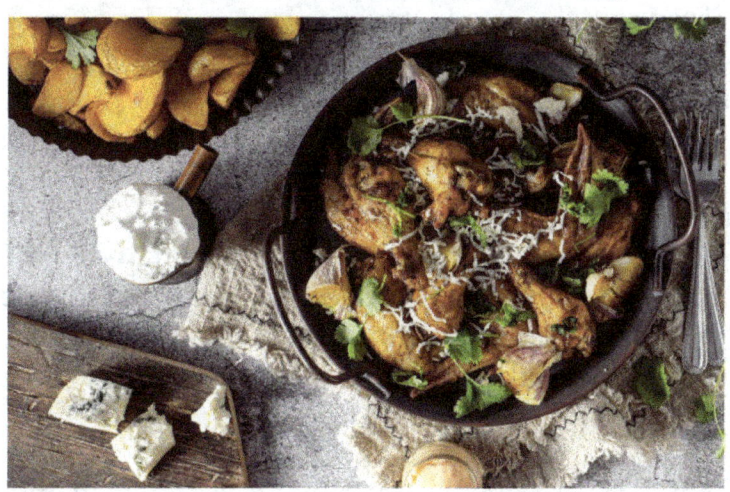

Servings: 4
4g 2% Net carbs
50g 24% Protein
67g 74% Fat
Total: 5 g
(kcal: 830)

Ingredients:

Blue-cheesedressing
- 1/3 cup mayonnaise
- ¼ cup sourcream
- 3 tsp lemonjuice
- ¼ tsp garlicpowder
- ¼ tsp salt
- ¼ cup heavy whippingcream
- 3 oz. blue cheese, crumbled

Chicken wings
- 2 lbs chicken wings
- 2 tbsp olive oil or melted bacon fat
- ¼ tsp garlicpowder
- 1 mincedgarlicclove

- ¼ tsp ground black pepper
- 1 tsp salt
- ½ cup (1⅓ oz.) shreddedParmesancheese

Serving
- 12 oz. (3⅓ cups) celerystalks

Instructions:
1. Use a whisk to stir together all of the ingredients for the dressing, except for the cheese. Once blended, add in blue cheese crumbles and mix well.
2. Chill for about 45 minutes before serving.

Chicken wings
3. Place the chicken in a large bowl. Add the oil and spices. Stir to coat the chicken. Marinate in the refrigerator for atleast 30 minutes.
4. Grill or bake in an oven at 425°F (200°C) for 30 minutes or until browned and crisp.
5. Place the baked wings in a large bowl and add the Parmesan cheese. Toss the wings in the cheeseuntilcoated.
6. Serve warm together with the dressing and celery stalks.

Instant Pot seafood bisque

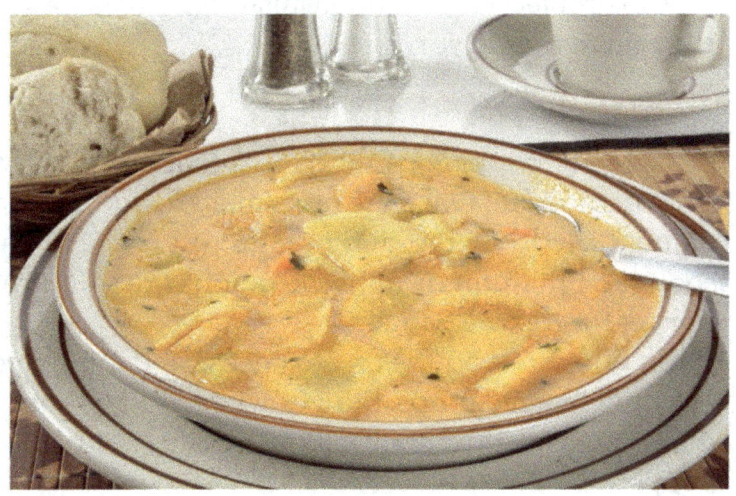

Servings: 6
6g 8% Net carbs
16g 22% Protein
24g 70% Fat
Total: 8 g
(kcal: 305)

Ingredients:

- 2 tbsp unsalted butter or coconut oil
- 1 (3 oz.) leek, trimmed, halved lengthwise, and sliced
- 1 (4 oz.) red onion, diced
- 1 (1½ oz.) celerystalk, diced
- 1 tsp freshthyme
- 1 tsp orangezest
- 8 oz. (1 cup) creamcheese, softened
- 3 cups chicken broth
- 2 tbsp tomato paste
- 1 tsp orangeextract (optional)
- 12 oz. shrimp, precooked
- 1 tsp salt
- ½ tsp ground black pepper

- 1 tbsp finely chopped fresh chives, for garnish
- 3 oz. crumbled bacon, for garnish
- 1 tsp olive oil, for garnish

Instructions:
1. Place the butter or coconut oil in a 6-quart Instant Pot and press Sauté. Once the fat is melted, add the leeks, onions, celery, thyme, and orange zest to the pot and cook for 4 minutes or until the onions are soft. Press Cancel to stop the Sauté.
2. Use a whisk to add the cream cheese and stir to loosen or you will get clumps. Slowly whisk in the broth. Add the tomato paste, orange extract, shrimp, salt, and pepper.
3. Seal the lid, press Pressure Cook or Manual, and set the timer for 2 minutes. Once finished, let the pressure release naturally.
4. Ladle the soup into bowls and garnish the bisque with chives and bacon. Drizzle with the olive oil.

Low-carb pâté with cranberry pickled red onions

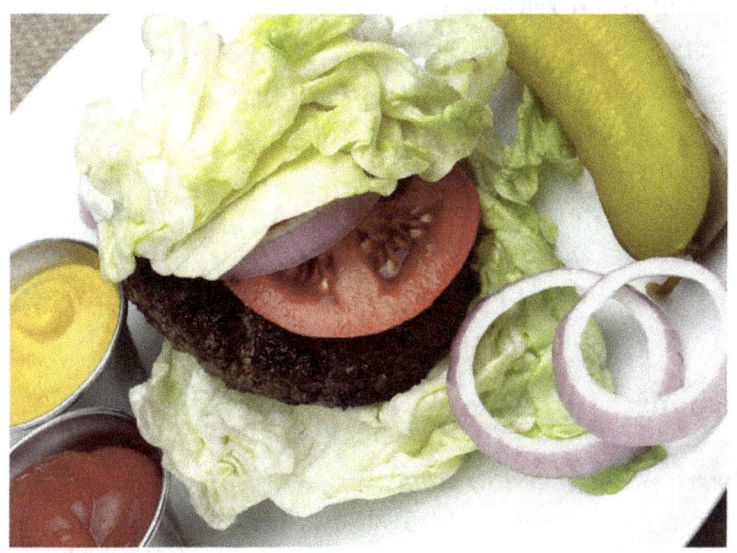

Servings: 12
3g 6% Net carbs
16g 34% Protein
13g 60% Fat
Total: 3 g
(kcal: 195)

Ingredients:

Cranberrypickled red onions
- 1 (4 oz.) red onion, thinlysliced
- ½ cup fresh or frozen cranberries or lingonberries
- ½ cup applecidervinegar
- ½ cup water
- ½ tsp salt

Christmas pâté
- 16 oz. chicken livers or beef liver, drained
- 8 oz. ground beef
- 6 oz. bacon
- 1 (1 oz.) shallot, finelychopped

- 15 driedjuniperberries
- 2 tsp freshrosemary
- 2 tsp salt
- 1 tsp ground black pepper
- 1 large egg
- 2/3 cup sourcream
- 2 tsp butter

For serving
- 3½ oz. dillpickles (optional)

Instructions:

Cranberry pickled red onions
1. In a medium-sized bowl, mix together red onions, cranberries, vinegar, water, and salt. Let marinate in the refrigerator for at least one day before serving.

Christmas pâté
2. Preheat the oven to 300°F (150°C). Cut the liver and bacon into small pieces. Place the liver, ground beef, bacon, and the chopped shallot in a food processor. Mix into a coarse batter.
3. Crush juniper berries and rosemary with a mortar and pestle or with a spice mill or coffee grinder until powdered. Add the juniper berries, rosemary, salt, and pepper, egg, and sour cream into the food processor. Mix a few seconds to combine.
4. Grease a loaf pan with butter. Pour the batter into the pan. Bake for 1 hour, covered with aluminum foil. Remove the foil and continue baking for an additional 15-20 minutes.

5. Remove from the oven and let cool for 10-15 minutes. Use a spatula to remove the pâté from the loaf pan and place it on a serving dish. Serve cooled to room temperature or wrap tightly and refrigerate before serving.
6. Slice the pâté and serve with pickled red onions and cranberries as well as dill pickles if desired.

Low-carb chicken dumplings

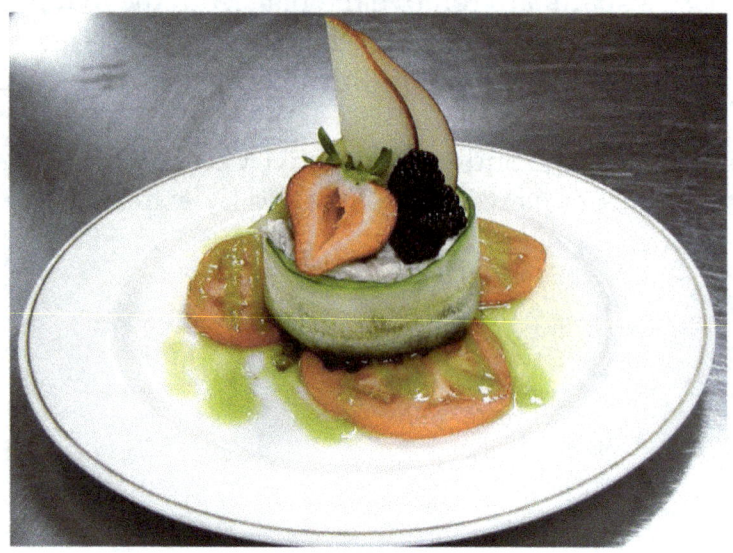

Servings: 5
6g 12% Net carbs
22g 41% Protein
11g 47% Fat
Total: 9 g
(kcal: 214)

Ingredients:

Dipping sauce
- 1 tsp peanutbutter
- 1 tsp srirachasauce
- ½ tsp ginger garlic paste
- ½ tsp tamari soysauce
- ½ tsp ricevinegar
- 1 tsp freshcilantro, chopped
- 1 tsp olive oil
- 1 pinch salt
- ½ lime, juiced

Chicken dumplings
- 1¼ lbs ground chicken
- 1 tsp salt
- ½ tsp Szechuanpepper
- ½ tsp pandanpowder (optional)
- ½ tsp cayenne pepper
- 1 tsp ginger garlic paste
- 1 (4 oz.) small red onion, grated
- ½ (¼ oz.) scallion
- 1 tsp freshcilantro, chopped
- 1 tbsp sesame oil (optional)
- 1 green cabbage (10 leaves)

Instructions:

Dippingsauce
1. Add peanut butter, sriracha sauce, ginger garlic paste, soy sauce, vinegar and cilantro in a small bowl. Mix untilcombinedthoroughly.
2. Add oil and mix well. Sprinkle with salt and lime juice. Combine well and set aside.

Chicken dumplings
3. Season ground chicken with salt, Szechuan pepper, pandan powder and cayenne pepper.
4. Add ginger garlic paste, grated red onion, scallion and cilantro. Mix well. Add sesame oil if you're using any and combine thoroughly.
5. Separate the cabbage leaves. In a large pot, boil in lightly salted water for 5-7 minutes until tender. Remove the leaves from the pot but keep the water simmering on low heat.
6. Stuff the individual cabbage leaves with the chicken filling and roll into dumplings.

7. Steam the dumplings for 10 minutes over the boiling water.
8. You can additionally fry the dumplings in a pan with a tablespoon of olive oil to get a golden crust.
9. Serve with dipping sauce and enjoy!

Low-carb salad olivieh

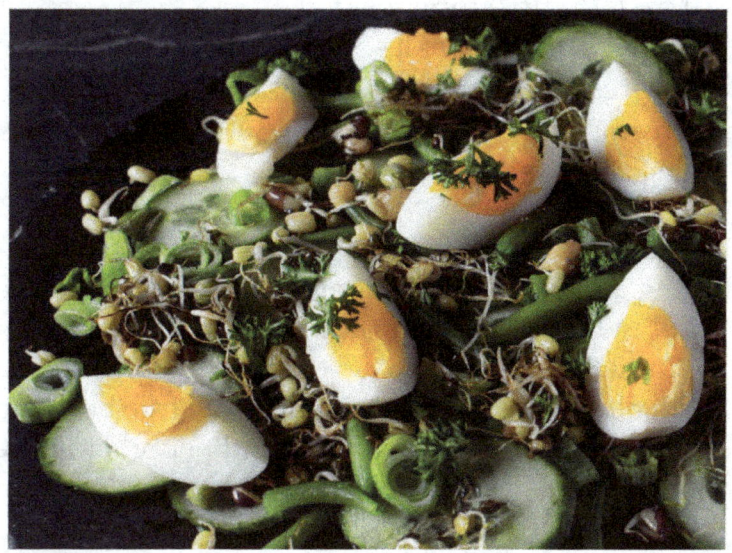

Servings: 12
7g 5% Net carbs
23g 14% Protein
57g 81% Fat
Total: 11 g
(kcal: 641)

Ingredients:

Salad
- 1¼ lbs rutabaga, peeled and diced
- 1¼ lbs mayonnaise
- 15 oz. sugar-free, dill pickles, diced
- 8 oz. frozen green peas, thawed
- 3½ oz. green olives, chopped
- 2 lbs rotisserie chicken, shredded
- 10 large, hard boiledeggs, chopped
- ¼ cup lemonjuice
- 2 tsp cayenne pepper
- salt and ground black pepper, to taste

Garnish
- 10 oz. (1½ cups) tomatoes
- 2 sugar-free, dill pickles, spears, cut into thirds
- 1 oz. fresh mint, minced, plus 1 sprig of mint
- 8 green olives, sliced
- 2 tbsp olive oil

Instructions
1. Bring a pot of salted water to a boil, over high heat. Add the diced rutabaga and boil for about 20 minutes, or until tender.
2. Add all of the salad ingredients to a large bowl, and mix together. Season with salt and pepper, to taste.
3. Spread the salad onto a large serving dish and garnish with the sliced tomatoes, sliced pickle, fresh mint, and olives. Drizzle with olive oil.
4. Enjoy immediately, or to maximize flavor refrigerate for 1 hour, or overnight.

Green gazpacho

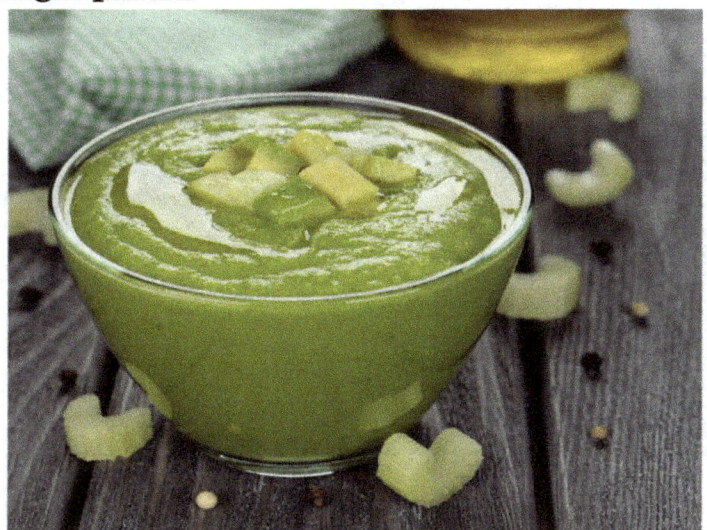

Servings: 3
10g 12% Net carbs
5g 7% Protein
30g 82% Fat
Total: 12 g
(kcal: 320)

Ingredients:

- 2½ oz. (½ cup) pre-soaked cashew nuts, drained
- ¾ cup (22/3 oz.) dicedcelerystalks
- 1 oz. (¾ cup) watercressleaves
- 3 oz. sliced cucumber, peeled and seeded
- 5 oz. Romainelettuce
- ¼ cup extra virgin olive oil
- 1 garlicclove
- 1 tsp fine salt
- 1 cup chicken broth or vegetable stock

Instructions:

1. Combine all of the ingredients in a blender and blend until smooth and creamy. Enjoyrightaway.

Low-carb guacamole

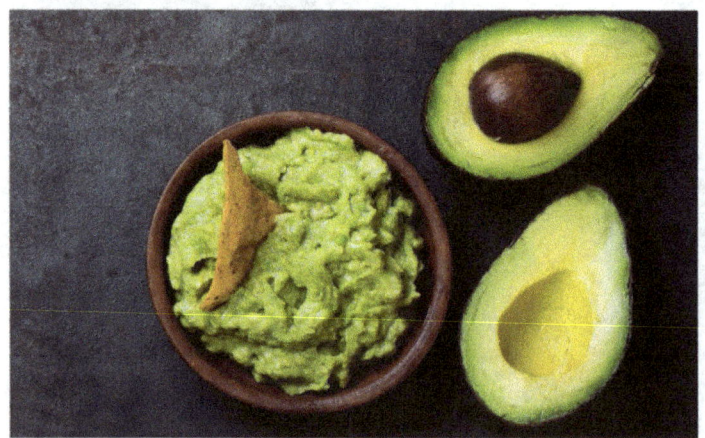

Servings: 4
5g 8% Net carbs
3g 5% Protein
21g 87% Fat
Total: 12 g
(kcal: 234)

Ingredients:
- 2 (14 oz.) ripe avocados
- ½ (2 oz.) white onion, grated or finely chopped
- ½ lime, the juice
- 1 (4 oz.) tomato, diced
- 2 tbsp olive oil
- ¼ cup (1⁄8 oz.) freshcilantro
- 1 garlicclove, minced
- salt and pepper, to taste

Instructions:
1. Peel the avocados and mash with a fork.
2. Add the onion, lime juice, tomato, olive oil, cilantro and garlic.
3. Season with salt and pepper, and mix until well combined.

Keto tortilla with ground beef and salsa

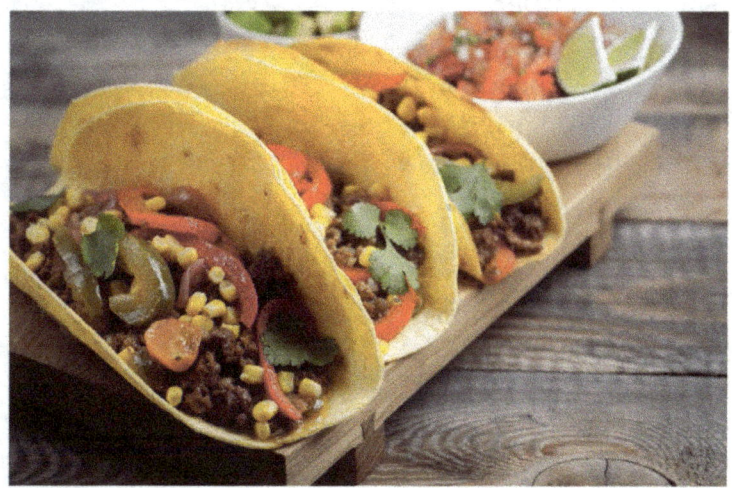

Servings: 4
7g 4% Net carbs
42g 21% Protein
68g 76% Fat
Total: 16 g
(kcal: 829)

Ingredients:

Low-carb tortillas
- 2 eggs
- 2 eggwhites
- 5 oz. (2/3 cup) creamcheese, softened
- ½ tsp salt
- 1½ tsp ground psylliumhuskpowder
- 1 tbsp coconutflour

Filling
- 2 tbsp olive oil
- 1 lb ground beef or ground turkey, at room temperature
- 2 tbsp Tex-Mex seasoning

- ½ cup water
- salt and pepper

Salsa
- 2 (14 oz.) avocados, diced
- 1 (4 oz.) tomato, diced
- 2 tbsp lime juice
- 1 tbsp olive oil
- ½ cup (¼ oz.) freshcilantro, chopped
- salt and pepper

For serving
- 1½ cups (6 oz.) shreddedMexicancheese
- 3 oz. (2⅓ cups) shreddedlettuce

Instructions:

Low-carb tortillas
1. Preheat the oven to 400°F (200°C).
2. Using an electric mixer with the whisk attachment, whisk the eggs and egg whites until fluffy, preferably for a few minutes. In a separate large bowl, beat the cream cheese until smooth. Add the eggs to the cream cheese, and whisk until the eggs and cream cheese form a smooth batter.
3. Mix salt, psyllium husk, and coconut flour in a small bowl. Add the flour mix one spoon at a time into the batter and continue to whisk some more. Let the batter sit for a few minutes, or until the batter is thick like an American pancake batter. How fast the batter will swell depends on the brand of psyllium husk – some trial and error might be needed.
4. Bring out two baking sheets and place parchment paper on each. Using a spatula, spread the batter thinly (no more than ¼ inch thick, 0.5cm) into 4–6 circles or 2 rectangles.

5. Bake on the upper rack for about 5 minutes or more, until the tortilla turns a little brown around the edges. Carefully check the bottom side so that it doesn't burn.

Filling
6. Place a large frying pan over medium-high heat and heat up the oil. Add the ground beef and fryuntilcookedthrough.
7. Add the tex-mex seasoning and water and stir. Let simmer until most of the water is gone. Taste to see if it needs additional seasoning.

Salsa and serving
8. Make the salsa from avocado, tomatoes, lime juice, olive oil, and fresh cilantro. Salt and pepper to taste.
9. Serve beef filling in a tortilla, with shredded cheese, salsa, and shredded leafy greens.

Low-carb tortillas

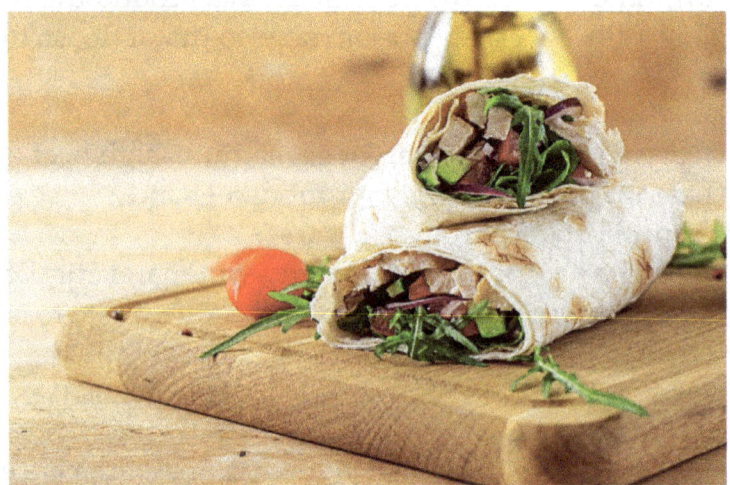

Servings: 6
2g 6% Net carbs
5g 17% Protein
10g 78% Fat
Total: 2 g
(kcal: 115)

Ingredients:

- 2 eggs
- 2 eggwhites
- 5 oz. (2/3 cup) creamcheese
- 1½ tsp ground psylliumhuskpowder
- 1 tbsp coconutflour
- ½ tsp salt

Instructions:

1. Preheat the oven to 400°F (200°C).
2. Beat the eggs and egg whites until fluffy. Continue to beat with a hand mixer, preferably for a few minutes. Add cream cheese and mix until the batter is smooth.

3. Mix salt, psyllium husk and coconut flour in a small bowl. Add the flour mixture to the batter one spoonful at a time and mix well. Let the batter sit for a few minutes, until it gets thick, like pancake batter. How quickly the batter swells depends on the brand of psyllium husk powder — some trial and error might be needed.
4. Bring out two baking sheets and place parchment paper on each. Using a spatula, spread the batter thinly (no more than ¼ inch thick) into 4–6 circles or 2 rectangles.
5. Bake on upper rack for about 5 minutes or more, until the tortilla turns a little brown around the edges. Carefully check the bottom side so that it doesn't burn.
6. Serve with a filling of your choice. We love them with tex-mex ground beef and salsa! And cheeseisalways a winner.

Keto quesadillas

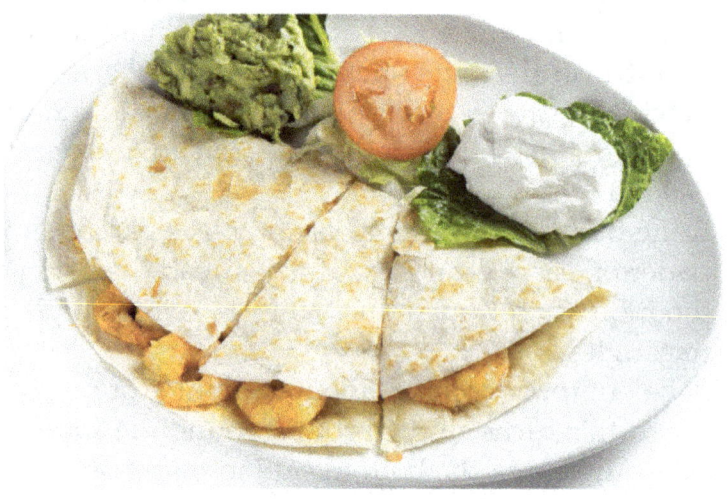

Servings: 3
4g 3% Net carbs
21g 18% Protein
42g 79% Fat
Total: 4 g
(kcal: 484)

Ingredients:
Low-carb tortillas
- 2 eggs
- 2 eggwhites
- 6 oz. (¾ cup) creamcheese
- ½ tsp salt
- 1½ tsp ground psylliumhuskpowder
- 1 tbsp coconutflour

Filling
- 1 tbsp olive oil or butter, for frying
- 5 oz. (1¼ cups) Mexican cheese or any hard cheese of your liking
- 1 oz. (1 cup) baby spinach

Instructions:

Tortillas
1. Preheat the oven to 400°F (200°C).
2. Using an electric mixer, beat eggs and egg whites together until fluffy. Add cream cheese and continue to beat until the batter is smooth.
3. In a bowl, combine salt, psyllium husk and coconut flour. Mix well.
4. Add the flour mixture into the batter while beating. When combined, let the batter sit for a few minutes. It should be thick like pancake batter. Your brand of psyllium husk powder affects this step — be patient... Ifitdoesnotthickenenough, add some more.
5. Place parchment paper on a baking sheet. Use a spatula to spread the batter over the parchment paper into a big rectangle. If you want round tortillas you can fry them in a frying pan like pancakes.
6. Bake on the upper rack for about 5–10 minutes, until the tortilla turns brown around the edges. Keep your eye on the oven — don't let these tasty creations burn on the bottom!
7. Cut the big tortilla into smaller pieces (6 pieces per baking sheet).

Quesadillas
8. Heat oil or butter in a small, non-stick skillet over medium heat.
9. Put a tortilla in the frying pan and sprinkle with cheese, spinach and with some more cheese. Top with another tortilla.
10. Fry each quesadilla for about a minute on each side. You'll know it's done when the cheese melts.

Soft keto tortillas

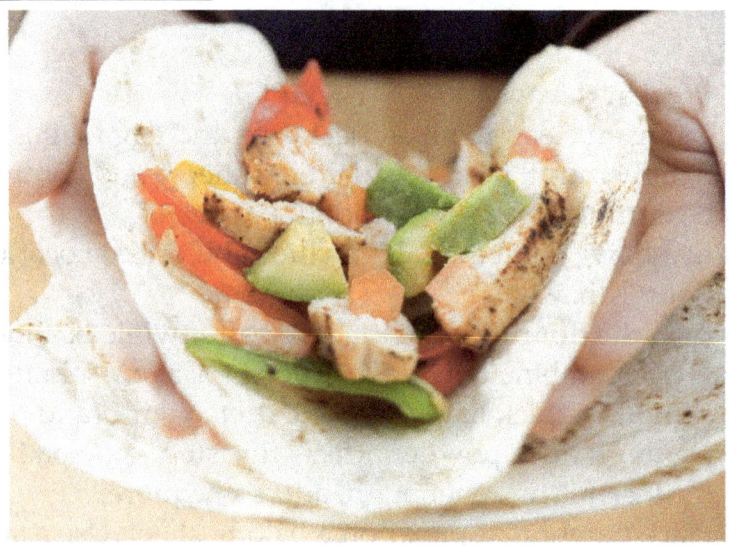

Servings: 6
1g 3% Net carbs
5g 9% Protein
21g 88% Fat
Total: 2 g
(kcal: 236)

Ingredients:
- 1 cup (31⁄3 oz.) coconutflour
- ¼ tsp baking soda
- ½ tsp salt
- ¼ cup (11⁄3 oz.) ground psyllium husk powder
- ½ cup avocado oil or olive oil
- 3 large eggwhites
- 1½ cups hot water

Instructions:
1. Heat a large cast iron skillet or griddle medium heat.
2. In a large bowl, sift together the coconut flour, baking soda and salt. Whisk in the psylliumhusk.
3. Drizzle in the oil slowly as you stir the mix, it will become moist and crumbly. Fold in the eggwhites.
4. Mix in the hot water half cup at a time, making sure it's completely mixed in before adding more water. Combine until the dough looks and feels like moist play-doh.
5. Shape 12 even-sized balls. Flatten the balls between parchment paper on a tortilla press or use a 6" pot and press them down.
6. Cook 2 tortillas at a time on the large griddle by lying flat on the hot, dry cast iron and toasting 3 minutes a side, flipping once. Set asideuntilall the tortillas are done.

Bacon-wrapped halloumi cheese

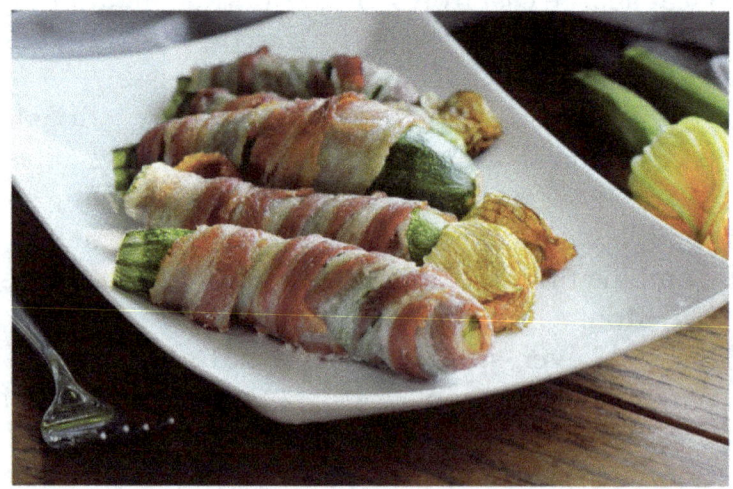

Servings: 2
4g 2% Net carbs
52g 28% Protein
57g 70% Fat
Total: 4 g
(kcal: 748)

Ingredients:
- 8 oz. halloumicheese
- 6 oz. bacon, in slices

Instructions:
1. Preheat the oven to 450°F (225°C).
2. Cutcheeseinto 8–10 pieces.
3. Wrap a piece of bacon around each piece of cheese.
4. Place on a baking sheet and bake in oven until golden brown for 10–15 minutes, flipping halfway through.

Keto egg muffins

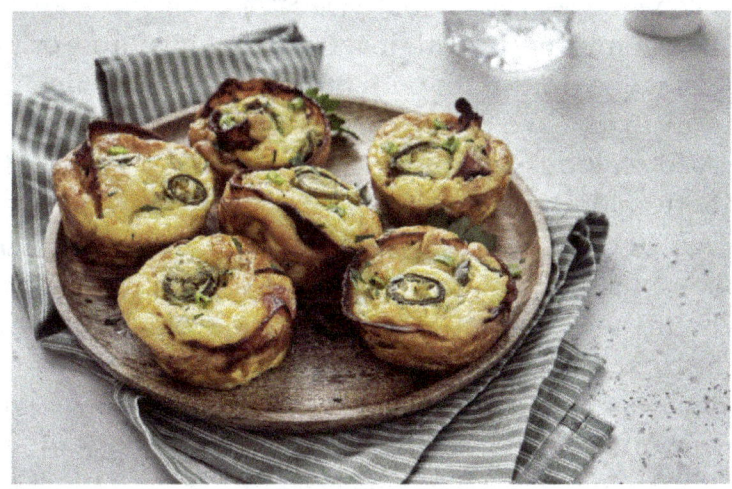

Servings: 6
2g 3% Net carbs
26g 30% Protein
26g 68% Fat
Total: 2 g
(kcal: 353)

Ingredients:

- 2 (1 oz.) scallions, finelychopped
- 5 oz. cooked bacon or salami, chopped
- 12 eggs
- 2 tbsp red pesto or green pesto (optional)
- salt and pepper, to taste
- 1½ cups (6 oz.) shredded cheddar cheese

Instructions:
1. Preheat the oven to 350°F (175°C).
2. Line a muffin tin with insertable baking cups, or grease a silicone muffin tin with butter, or use a non-stick muffin tin (two muffins per serving).
3. Add scallions and the cooked bacon or salami, to the bottom of the tin.
4. Whisk together the eggs, pesto, salt, and pepper, until combined.
5. Pour the egg mixture on top of the scallions and meat. Sprinkle the cheese on top.
6. Bake for 15–20 minutes, depending on the size of the muffin tin.

Keto jalapeño popper chaffles

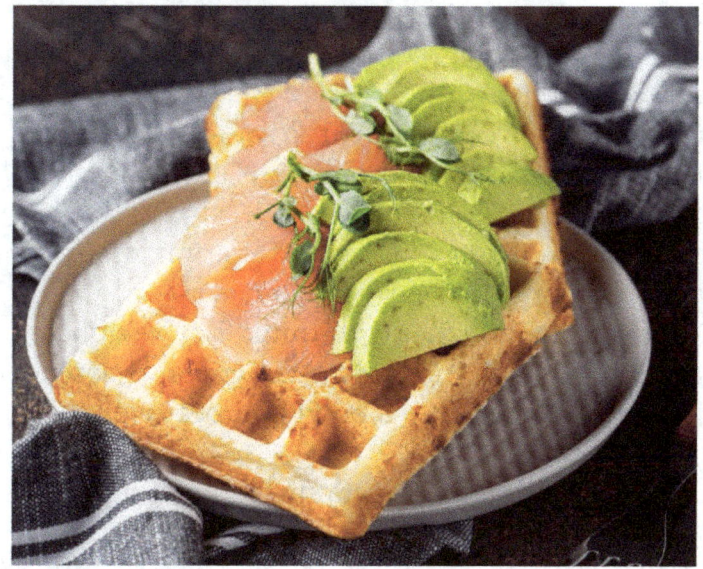

Servings: 4
5g 4% Net carbs
28g 22% Protein
40g 74% Fat
Total: 5 g
(kcal: 494)

Ingredients:

Chaffles
- 4 eggs
- 2 cups (8 oz.) shredded cheddar cheese
- 2 tbsp fresh chives, chopped (save some for garnish)

Topping
- ½ cup (4 oz.) creamcheese, softened
- ½ tsp garliccloves, minced
- 1 (½ oz.) scallion, choppedfinely
- 3 oz. bacon, chopped and cooked
- 2 freshjalapeños, seeded and sliced
- ½ (¼ oz.) scallion, chopped for garnish

Instructions:
1. Pre-heat your waffle maker.
2. Place all of your ingredients into a mixing bowl and beat to combine.
3. Lightly grease your waffle iron and then evenly spoon the mixture over the bottom plate, spreading it out slightly to get an even result.
4. Close the waffle iron and cook for approx 6 minutes, depending on your waffle maker.
5. Gently lift the lid when you think they're done.
6. While the waffles cook, place the cream cheese, garlic and spring onions into a bowl and beat well to combine.
7. Add most of the bacon, retaining some for garnish and stir through.
8. When waffles are ready, top with a big spoonful of cream cheese, sliced jalapeño to taste and the remaining chopped chives and bacon.

Keto eggs on the go

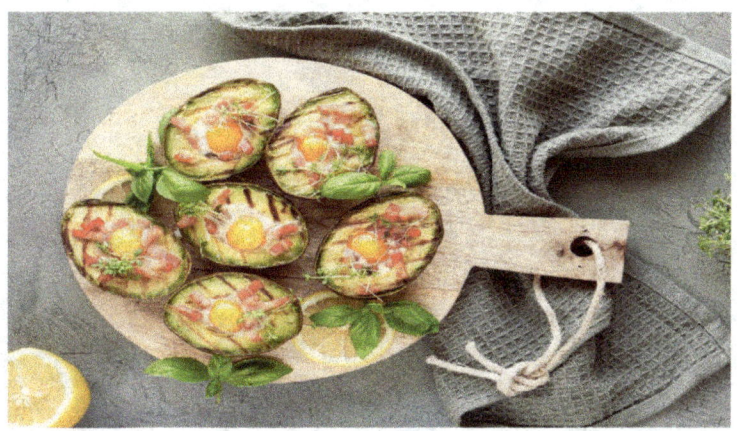

Servings: 6
1g 2% Net carbs
21g 33% Protein
18g 65% Fat
Total: 1 g
(kcal: 255)

Ingredients:
- 12 large eggs
- salt and pepper, to taste
- 5 oz. cooked bacon

Instructions:
1. Preheat the oven to 400°F (200°C).
2. Place cupcake liners in a muffin tin. Eggs easily stick even to non-stick surfaces, except for silicon forms.
3. Crack one egg in each form and add the filling of your choice. Choose one of our fillings below, or invent your own! We'regoing for classiccrumbled bacon.
4. Season to taste.
5. Bake in the oven for about 15 minutes or until the eggs are cooked.

Keto cheese roll-ups

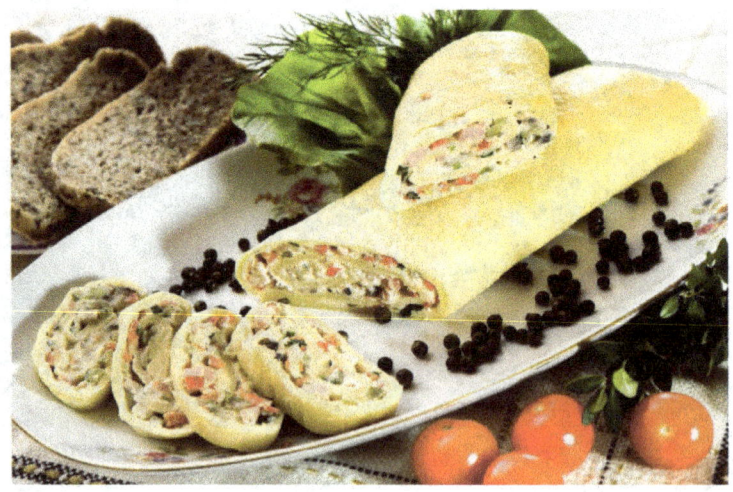

Servings: 4
 2g 2% Net carbs
13g 16% Protein
30g 82% Fat
Total: 2 g
(kcal: 330)

Ingredients:
- 8 oz. (2 cups) cheddar cheese or provolone cheese or edam cheese, in slices
- 2 oz. butter

Instructions:
1. Place the cheese slices on a large cutting board.
2. Slice butter with a cheese slicer or cut really thin pieces with a knife.
3. Cover every cheese slice with butter and roll up. Serve as a snack.

Keto bresaola plate

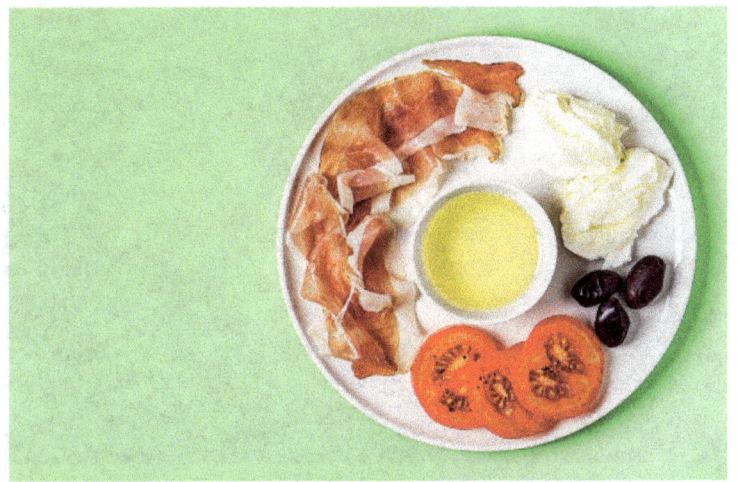

Servings: 4
3g 2% Net carbs
27g 22% Protein
41g 75% Fat
Total: 3 g
(kcal: 494)

Ingredients:
- 2 oz. bresaola, thinlysliced
- 1 oz. parmesancheese, thinlysliced
- 1 cup (2/3 oz.) arugulalettuce
- 1 boiled large egg, cut in half
- 1 tbsp freshlemonjuice
- 2 tbsp olive oil
- salt and pepper to taste

Instructions:
1. Layout the bresaola on the plate.
2. Top with arugula, parmesan cheese, and egg.
3. Drizzle with olive oil, lemon juice, and add salt and pepper to taste.

Stuffed mini bell peppers

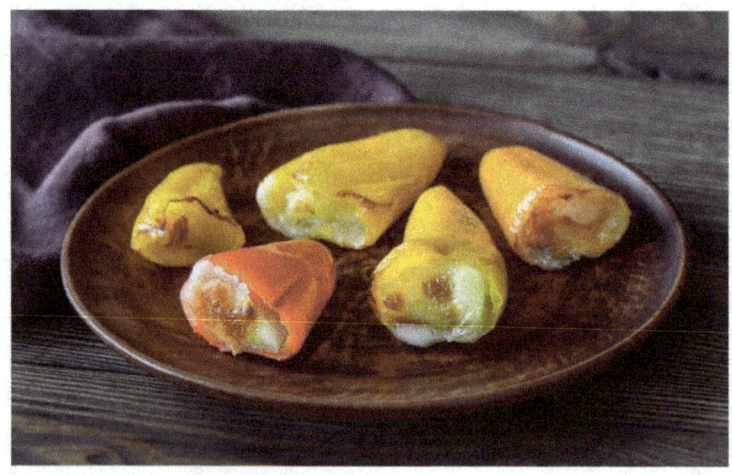

Servings: 4
9g 11% Net carbs
7g 8% Protein
29g 81% Fat
Total: 12 g
(kcal: 334)

Ingredients:
- 8 mini bellpeppers
- 8 oz. (1 cup) cream cheese, room temperature
- 1 oz. hard salami, thinly sliced and chopped finely
- ½ tbsp mildchipotle paste
- 2 tbsp olive oil
- 1 tbsp fresh thyme or fresh cilantro, chopped finely

Instructions:
1. Slice the peppers in half, lengthwise. Using a small spoon, remove the seeds and ribs.
2. In a small bowl, mix together the cream cheese, salami, chipotle paste, olive oil, and herbs, until well combined.
3. Stuff the peppers with the cream cheese mixture, and serve as a snack or an appetizer.

Low-carb eggplant pizza

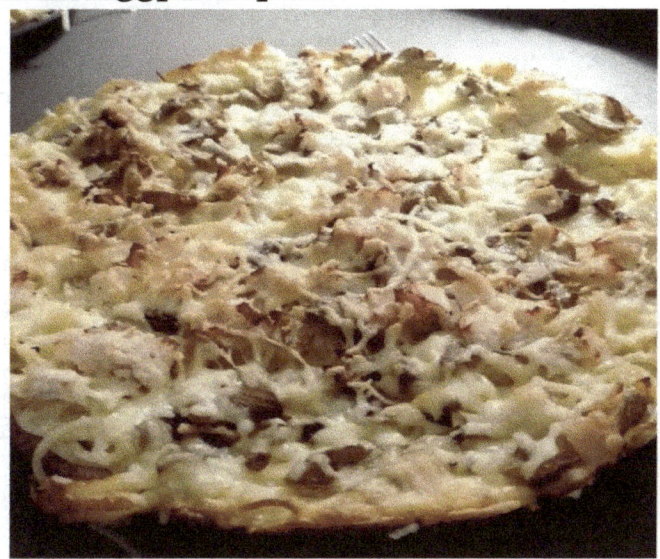

Servings: 4
13g 9% Net carbs
36g 24% Protein
45g 67% Fat
Total: 22 g
(kcal: 625)

Ingredients:
- 2 (2¼ lbs) eggplant
- 1/3 cup olive oil, for brushing and frying
- 2 garliccloves, minced
- 1 (4 oz.) yellowonion, choppedfinely
- ¾ lb ground beef or ground turkey
- ¾ cup sugar-free tomato sauce
- 1 tsp salt
- ½ tsp pepper
- ½ tsp ground cinnamon (optional)
- 2½ cups (10 oz.) mozzarella cheese, shredded
- ¼ cup choppedfreshoregano

Instructions:
1. Preheat the oven to 400°F (200°C).
2. Slice the eggplants lengthwise, about ⅓–½ inches (1 cm) thick. Coat with olive oil on both sides and place on a baking sheet lined with parchment paper.Bake for about 20 minutes or untilslightlybrowned.
3. Fry garlic and onion in remaining olive oil until softened, about 3-4 minutes.
4. Add beef and sauté until cooked through. Add tomato sauce, and season with salt and pepper. Letsimmer for 10 minutes, or untilwarmedthrough.
5. Remove the eggplant slices from the oven and spread the meat mixture on top. Sprinkle with cheese and oregano. Place in the oven for about 10 minutes or until the cheese has melted.
6. Serve with a green salad dressed with olive oil.

Keto pizza crust

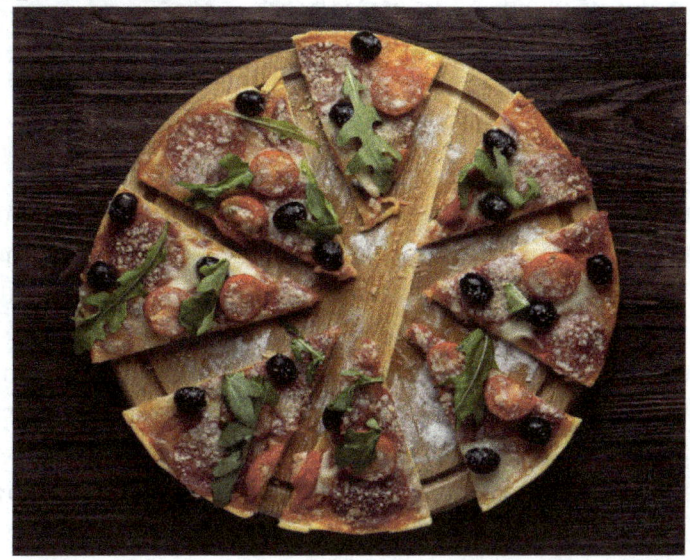

Servings: 4
3g 3% Net carbs
17g 19% Protein
31g 78% Fat
Total: 3 g
(kcal: 384)

Ingredients:
- 1¼ cups (5 oz.) almondflour
- ¼ cup unflavoredproteinpowder
- ¼ cup (11/3 oz.) ground psyllium husk powder
- ½ tsp salt
- 2 tbsp gratedparmesancheese
- 1 tbsp Italianseasoning
- 2 tsp bakingpowder
- 2 eggs
- 1 cup boiling water
- 1½ oz. melted butter or coconut oil, for brushing
- olive oil for greasing

Instructions

1. Preheat the oven to 350°F (176°C). Line two baking sheets with parchment paper, or use non-stick baking sheets, and lightly coat either option with olive oil.
2. In a medium-sized bowl, mix the dry ingredients together. Add the eggs, and stir until combined.
3. Slowly add boiling water to the mixture, and mix until the dough thickens, and becomes sticky. Divide the dough in half. Lightly moisten hands with olive oil, and shape the dough into two balls.
4. Put each ball in the center of the baking sheets, topped with a touch of olive oil. Place parchment papers on top of each ball. Lay a rolling pin, or your hands on top of the parchment papers, to shape and flatten the dough into two, 10-inch (25 cm) round, thin crusts. Discard the upper parchment papers. Using a fork, prick holes all over the crusts to help prevent bubbles from forming.
5. Bake on the middle rack(s) for about 20-25 minutes, or until lightly browned.
6. Remove, and brush with butter or coconut oil.
7. Increase the temperature to the Broil setting (Watch closely during this step to make sure that the crusts become crispy, yet not burnt). Broil both sides of the pizza base until light brown and crispy, approximately 1-3 minutes per side.
8. Set aside to cool, and then store in the freezer until you want to use them. If you can't wait, pre-heat the oven to 425 °F (218°C), add toppings and bake on the middle rack for 5-10 minutes, or until the cheese is melted, and starts to brown.

Low-carb cauliflower pizza with artichokes

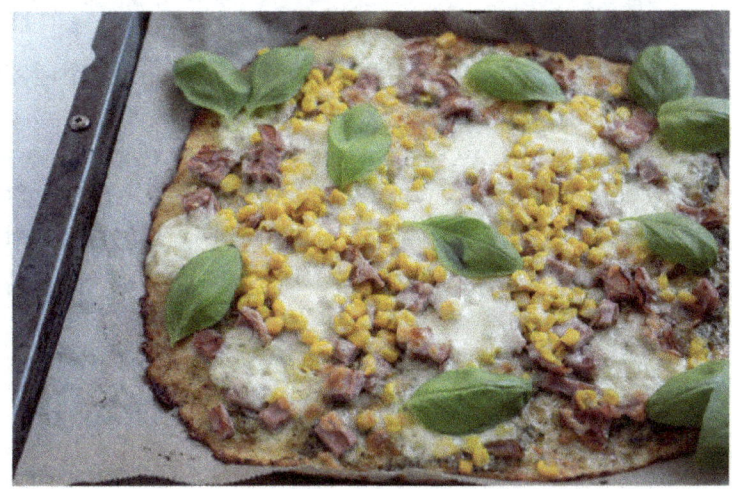

Servings: 1
14g 6% Net carbs
66g 29% Protein
65g 65% Fat
Total: 21 g
(kcal: 935)

Ingredients:

Crust
- 1 cup (4 oz.) shredded mozzarella cheese
- 5 oz. cauliflower
- 2 large eggs
- ½ tsp salt

Pizza toppings
- 2 tbsp tomato sauce, unsweetened
- ½ cup (2 oz.) shredded cheddar cheese
- ½ cup (2 oz.) shredded mozzarella cheese
- 2 oz. canned artichokes, drained and cut into wedges
- 1 tbsp dried oregano or finely chopped, fresh basil
- 1 garlic clove, thinly sliced (optional)

Instructions:

Crust
1. Preheat the oven to 350°F (180°C). Line a baking sheet with parchment paper.
2. Grate the cauliflower using a food processor or a grater. Place the cauliflower, mozzarella cheese, and eggs into a medium-sized bowl and stir together, until combined.
3. Using a spatula, spread the mixture on the baking sheet, forming a circular, thin-crust, about 11" (28 cm) in diameter. Bake on the middle rack for about 20 minutes, or until lightly browned. Set aside.

Pizza
4. Raise the oven temperature to 420°F (210°C). Spread the tomato sauce over the crust, and then layer with the mozzarella cheese, artichokes, basil, oregano, and garlic on top.
5. Bake on the middle rack for 5-10 minutes, or until the crust and cheese turn golden brown. Slice and enjoy!

CPSIA information can be obtained
at www.ICGtesting.com
Printed in the USA
BVHW090536220621
610124BV00011B/2495